Passing the **UKCAT** and **BMAT**

2012 Edition

Felicity Taylor, Rosalie Hutton and Glenn Hutton

Seventh edition

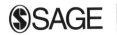

Los Angeles | London | New Delhi
Singapore | Washington DC

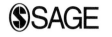

Learning Matters
An imprint of SAGE Publications Ltd
1 Oliver's Yard
55 City Road
London EC1Y 1SP

SAGE Publications Inc.
2455 Teller Road
Thousand Oaks, California 91320

SAGE Publications India Pvt Ltd
B 1/I 1 Mohan Cooperative Industrial Area
Mathura Road
New Delhi 110 044

SAGE Publications Asia-Pacific Pte Ltd
3 Chuch Street
#10–04 Samsung Hub
Singapore 049483

Editor: Amy Thornton
Development Editor: Jennifer Clark
Production Controller: Chris Marke
Project Management: Deer Park Productions,
Tavistock
Marketing Manager: Catherine Slinn
Cover Design: Toucan
Typeset by: Pantek Media, Maidstone, Kent
Printed by: MPG Books Group, Bodmin, Cornwall

FSC

First published in 2006
Reprinted in 2006 (twice)
Second edition published in 2007
Reprinted in 2007 (three times)
Third edition published in 2008
Reprinted in 2008 (twice)
Fourth edition published in 2009
Reprinted in 2009
Fifth edition published in 2010
Reprinted in 2010
Sixth edition published in 2011
Reprinted in 2011
Seventh edition published in 2012

Library of Congress Control Number: 2012931685

British Library Cataloguing in Publication Data

A catalogue record for this book is available from the
British Library

ISBN: 978 0 85725 867 0
ISBN: 978 0 85725 777 2 (pbk)

Passing the **UKCAT** and **BMAT**

Seventh edition

Contents

Part II: Preparing for the UK Clinical Aptitude Test (UKCAT) 49

Rosalie Hutton and Glenn Hutton

Part III: Preparing for the BioMedical Admissions Test (BMAT)

215

Felicity Taylor

Acknowledgements

The publisher and authors would like to thank the following for permission to reproduce extracts:

The British Psychological Society – Extract from Patrick Packwood, 'Enabling dyslexics to cope in employment' (2006) *Selection & Development Review* 22(1).

Guardian Newspapers Limited – Extract from Randeep Ramesh, 'Drug firms seek to stop generic HIV treatment', 11 May 2006.

Oxford University Press – Extract from Fraser Sampson, Blackstone's Police Manual, Volume 4, *General Police Duties* (2005).

Every effort has been made to contact copyright holders for their permission to reproduce extracts contained in this book. Apologies are offered for any errors or omissions, which will be rectified in future editions.

FT: To my parents and Damian

RH and GH: To the memory of Martin Orme

Part I
Introduction

Chapter 1
Introduction to the tests

As competition for university places continues to increase, admissions tutors are requiring more detailed assessment of students applying to university, in order to best discover their suitability for studying at undergraduate level. Nowhere has this extra burden of assessment been felt more keenly than in applying to read medicine, dentistry and veterinary science/medicine: due to the huge numbers of high-quality applicants competing for each available place, with often nothing to choose between candidates in terms of exam results, the schools have turned towards alternative methods of assessing candidates' aptitudes. The first test to come into existence was the BioMedical Admissions Test (BMAT), which combines aptitude tests with an assessment of scientific knowledge and reasoning skills. At the five medical and veterinary schools that currently use the BMAT, it has proved very successful in providing a more in-depth description of candidates' strengths and weaknesses, allowing admissions tutors to use this information as part of their selection process.

The second test that has been developed is the UK Clinical Aptitude Test (UKCAT). The UKCAT aims to test verbal reasoning, quantitative reasoning, abstract reasoning and decision analysis rather than scientific knowledge. Unlike its cousin the BMAT, the UKCAT has been taken up by the majority of UK medical schools and some dentistry schools, so it is likely that, if you are intending to apply to university to read medicine or dentistry, you will have to sit the UKCAT. Although now well established, the UKCAT continues to create a large amount of anxiety. Some candidates will have to sit both the BMAT and UKCAT and may feel unsure how they will manage to prepare for both tests while still keeping up with their normal studies.

This book has been fully updated and has been designed to assist you to prepare for both the BMAT and UKCAT exams by helping you to familiarise yourself with the types of questions used, and how to solve them. The developers of both the BMAT and UKCAT advise that their tests cannot be revised for, but it is certain that they can definitely be prepared for: a familiarity with what you will meet in the test and a knowledge of what is required of you, combined with confidence in answering the questions, will enable you to fulfil your full potential and will remove a lot of the unnecessary anxiety and stress these tests generate.

Part I of this book contains advice and practical support on applying to medical school, taking you through the application process step by step, including details on how to write your personal statement, how to arrange work experience and how to succeed in interviews.

In Part II of this book you will find detailed instructions on how to prepare for the UKCAT exam, including analysis of the types of questions you will encounter, practice tests and worked examples so that you can understand where mistakes are made and how to avoid them yourself. Additional questions have been added to this 7th edition.

Finally, Part III tackles the BMAT, providing examples and exam-style tests so that you can familiarise yourself with the standard required and build your confidence prior to the test. In this part there is also a detailed discussion regarding the essay section, with tips on how to research, plan and write the perfect essay.

While this book cannot promise you a guaranteed pass on the UKCAT and BMAT, if you follow the advice it offers and practise the questions it contains, we can promise that you will be much better prepared for the tests – which will permit you to achieve your best possible result.

All about the tests

The following text provides you with all the general and administrative information regarding the UK Clinical Aptitude Test (UKCAT) and the Biomedical Admissions Test (BMAT).

Who needs to sit the tests?

UKCAT

University of Aberdeen	A100, A201
Barts and the London School of Medicine and Dentistry	A100, A101, A200, A201
Brighton and Sussex Medical School	A100
Cardiff University	A100, A104, A200, A204
University of Dundee	A100, A104, A200, A204
University of Durham	A100
University of East Anglia	A100, A104
University of Edinburgh	A100
University of Glasgow	A100, A200
Hull York Medical School	A100
Imperial College London Graduate Entry	A101
Keele University	A100, A104

King's College London	A100, A101, A102, A202, A205
University of Leeds	A100
University of Leicester	A100, A101
University of Manchester	A104, A106, A204, A206
University of Newcastle	A100, A101, A206
University of Nottingham	A100, A108
University of Oxford Graduate Entry	A101
Peninsula College of Medicine and Dentistry	A100
Queen's University Belfast	A100, A200
University of Sheffield	A100, A104, A200
University of Southampton	A100, A101, A102
University of St Andrews	A100, A990, B900
St George's, University of London	A100
Warwick University Graduate Entry	A101

Plus applicants from other countries: check www.ukcat.ac.uk for details.

BMAT

University of Cambridge	A100, A101 (not essential), D100
Imperial College London	
(University of London)	A100, B900, B9N2
University of Oxford	A100 BC98
Royal Veterinary College	D100, D101, D102
University College London	A100

When are the tests?

BMAT – Wednesday 7 November 2012.
UKCAT – 3 July to 5 October 2012.

All about the UKCAT

Introduced in 2006, the UKCAT is an aptitude test designed to assess whether or not you have the appropriate professional attitude, mental abilities and problem-solving skills that will be necessary for a successful career in medicine or dentistry. It's used by a selection of medical schools as part of the application procedure (i.e. they look at your personal statement, your predicted grades and your teacher reference too) and they may use it to help to decide whether to call you for interview or offer you a place.

So as you can see from all the universities that require it, you're probably going to have to sit the UKCAT. The need for the UKCAT has arisen mainly out of the continuing increase in immensely well-qualified candidates applying for medicine, leaving admissions tutors with little to distinguish one candidate from another. The UKCAT does not include any questions that require science or A-level knowledge: think of it like an IQ or mental ability test. However, like anything in life, practice makes perfect, and you'll probably want to practise the types of questions likely to come up. You can look at the ones on the website (www.ukcat.ac.uk) and also use all the ones in this book.

In terms of the test administration, all the details can be found on the website, but in brief you will have to register online to take the test between 1 May 2012 and 21 September 2012 (for 2013 and deferred 2014 entry). You can sit the test any time you want between 3 July and 5 October (I would advise registering and booking a slot early, as the later dates get booked up quickly). The fee is around £65 if you sit the test before 31 August (£100 for overseas students); after this the fee jumps to £80. Bursaries will be available for those in financial need (make sure you apply via the website before you register to sit the test). There is also a version of the test, the UKCATSEN, which provides additional time for candidates with disabilities or medical conditions.

You will sit the test at a registered centre using a computer, and in total it will take just over 90 minutes. Each UKCAT subtest is separately timed, meaning you cannot overrun on one area and make it up in another. Results are available immediately, in theory enabling you to take your result into consideration before you have to submit your UCAS application form. However, there is no clear guidance available as to what constitutes a 'good' score, so I would consider it wise to see your result as part of your assessment and continue with your application to medical or dental school whatever the result. Please note, in 2011 sub-test 5 (behavioural traits) was discontinued.

There is no negative marking, and the computer will automatically scale your correct responses to give you a score between 300 and 900 in each of the first four subtests. In the past, the national average has been in the range of 2,400–2,500. UKCAT passes your score to the universities who require it and they use it as part of your admission assessment, along with your GCSE and A level grades and your personal statement.

Unfortunately there is no universal magic score on the UKCAT that guarantees an interview or a university place, although many universities use the same cut-off, below which you would not be considered further. For example, St Andrew's School of Medicine states on their website that candidates with a score less than a predetermined cut-off between 2,400 and 2,500 will not be considered for interview, although a score above this does not guarantee interview or entry. They then use your UKCAT score for ranking candidates post interview, making up 15 per cent of your admissions score. Other universities give similar advice, but most just state that the UKCAT test is required without providing any further advice on score. In these circumstances it would seem sensible to continue with your application as planned.

All *about* the BMAT

The BMAT is a little older than its cousin, the UKCAT. It has been around for a number of years and is required for students applying to the medicine, veterinary medicine and related courses such as pharmacology listed on page 5.

The BMAT consists of three sections, and is a paper exam sat at your school or local test centre. You'll sit this in November, so it shouldn't clash with the UKCAT. The first paper tests problem-solving and analysing arguments; the second tests your science and maths knowledge; and the third tests your ability to create structured, coherent arguments in an essay format. All the information you need regarding the test, including practice papers, sample answers and arrangements for sitting the test, is available on the BMAT website (www.admissionstests.cambridgeassessment.org.uk/adt/) which should be your first point of call for all your test queries. A point to note is that the entrance fee rises by £30 for late entries, so apply before 1 October 2012.

I personally think that there's a lot you can do to prepare for the BMAT, which is why you will find a detailed section later in this book telling you just how to approach the questions and with lots of examples for you to practise. Before the UKCAT came along, students used to get very stressed over the idea of the BMAT, but now you have the UKCAT to worry about too.

Oxford, Cambridge, UCL and Imperial all have a reputation among students as being 'hard' to get into, and by allowing themselves to have a different test from all the other medical schools they probably haven't helped their cause any. But the BMAT is a sensible test once you get the hang of it, so don't let it put you off applying to those universities.

Courses *not requiring* tests

Some of you may have noticed that there are a few medical schools offering standard entry courses which require neither the BMAT nor the UKCAT (for reasons unknown to us mere mortals). These are the University of Birmingham, the University of Bristol, the University of Liverpool and Queen Mary's, University of London. Some among you may now be hatching a plan for an application which requires no tests by applying to these medical schools. I wouldn't advise you to go down that route, mainly because these schools are likely to have lots of people applying to them as an 'insurance' place in case they fail the UKCAT, and so they may already be extra-competitive to get into. Additionally, there isn't much point in applying to a medical school you don't particularly want to go to merely to avoid a test which, with a bit of work, you can ace anyway.

Instead of thinking about the tests as a negative part of your application, look at them as having the potential to help you. The very fact you own this book indicates that you are committed to lots of hard work and preparation for the BMAT/UKCAT. If this is the case, then your test result will actually give you an advantage over everyone else, rather than it hampering your application. Just be sure to follow the advice and practise the questions in the second and third parts of this book.

Time management for the BMAT and UKCAT

By reading this book you will begin to understand the style and scope of the UKCAT and BMAT examination questions, and will hopefully realise that most of the questions do not present an intellectual challenge greater than that of your A-level courses. This is not to say that the exams are a walkover: the difficulty of these tests comes from the fact that the time allowed for their completion is extremely short, and that each of the subtests is individually timed and scored, preventing you from making up for lost time in areas of the test which you find easier. Until you have taken some mock examinations you won't really appreciate how difficult it is to answer all of the questions in the time available, and you certainly won't have much time (if any) for checking your answers. So throughout your preparation for the UKCAT and BMAT you need to focus on working accurately under time pressure and improving your performance in your weakest parts of the papers. Every year, even the most diligent students emerge from the examination room feeling that the exam was more difficult than they had expected and anxious that they didn't manage to complete or check all of their answers to the best of their ability. This is the challenge of the UKCAT and BMAT exams, and it is helpful to think of this situation as a mark of a successful examination method rather than a failure of the candidate. After all, there isn't much point taking an extra examination if there is no scope for stretching the very best students.

Below are a number of suggestions to help you to prepare yourself for the time pressure you will encounter in the UKCAT and BMAT examinations: as always, adequate preparation and practice will help to increase your confidence and alleviate much of the anxiety and stress of the exams.

Attempt practice papers with 10 per cent less time allowance

It is much less stressful doing a practice paper sitting in your bedroom with the cat in your lap and a plate of chocolate digestives within easy reach than it is doing the real thing in a cold school assembly hall with 40 other stressed-out candidates. To take account of this panic factor, always give yourself 10 per cent less time when you are doing the practice papers than you will be allowed for the real thing: hopefully by the time you get to the real exam you will be so efficient that you can use this 'free time' for checking or re-attempting tricky questions.

Attempt the practice papers 'blind'

Often it is tempting to have a look through the practice papers before you actually have a go at them: if you do this then your brain becomes familiar with the problems and may even start to solve them subconsciously before you actually come to sit the paper, hence the time pressure feels less acute. In short, it is easy to answer a question once you have seen it before (and may even have half-glanced at the answer while looking at another solution).

Have an order

The biggest cause of panic for most students is when turning over the paper and feeling they can't answer the first question, or the second, or the fifth, tenth, etc. This triggers a spiral of panic which can be extremely costly time-wise. Having a set order to how you tackle the paper really assists in helping you to achieve a sense of control. Whether you attempt the questions in the order they come, take the biology questions first in the BMAT or tackle the hardest/longest ones first/last in the UKCAT subsections, always keep this same order when practising sample papers and then you won't feel so phased in the exam room when you come across a tough first question.

Become a confident guesser

The fact that there is no negative marking on the BMAT and UKCAT means that even if you haven't a clue as to the answer, then you have approximately a 20 per cent chance of getting it right. That means, in a trade-off between spending the dying seconds of the exam trying to work out a complex bit of algebra, or answering an easy question and guessing a hard one, then it's worth a guess every time. This feels very strange for students used to carefully working out each answer, but the exams are constructed so as to allow for intelligent guesswork. This is something that you can practise with sample papers: never look up the answer to a question you can't do until you've made a guess at it – you will find in time that you develop a sixth sense for canny guesses.

Use the clock

In the actual UKCAT test you have a handy timer which starts counting down at the start of every section. With each section individually timed, you know exactly how much you have left. Don't be put off by the ticking clock; try to ignore it while answering each question, but do glance at it from time to time so you know when you have one or two minutes left. You won't have the time to go back to check your answers, but if things are getting tight you can at least have the time to make guesses on the last few questions rather than be timed out.

Read the instructions

Make sure that when you answer questions you do not lose marks by failing to read the question properly. In the BMAT marks are often lost by students failing to mark 'all that apply'. In the UKCAT the instructions for that question can be found in the bottom left of the screen, e.g. 'select the best response'.

Resources

You'll find practice questions for the UKCAT in Part II of this book, and practice questions for the BMAT in Part III. Included below is a selection of links that previous students have found useful. Remember, however, that these tests are only part of your application, and you shouldn't neglect your studies or your extracurricular activities for test revision, as these attributes are just as important to your application.

UKCAT

www.ukcat.ac.uk – specimen questions are available on the website, and you are strongly advised to do the online familiarity tutorial which provides a mock-up of how the computer test will look and operate. You can also see reports of past years' results.

www.onexamination.com/ukcat/ – offers limited practice questions to entice you to buy its question bank. Offers a one-month access package for around £26. Some students who want more practice find it useful.

BMAT

www.admissionstest.cambridgeassessment.org.uk.adt.bmat – this website has been updated and is much easier to use than previously. They have a specimen and past paper for each of the test sections, complete with answers and explanations. They also have examples of the answer papers, which it is good to familiarise yourself with. Also, an interesting piece of research from 2005 which shows your chance of getting a first at Cambridge based on your BMAT score.

www.ucl.ac.uk/lapt/bmat/ – an excellent free resource from UCL with a fair number of BMAT-style questions. It also gives you the answers as you go along. Just be aware that the 'confidence' rating to your answers isn't part of the actual test.

Good luck with the tests and your future career.

Chapter 2

So just why do you want to be a doctor?

This chapter will help you to:

- consider why you want to study at medical school;
- consider why you want a career as a doctor.

Congratulations – you've decided to choose a career in medicine. 'So, just why do you want to be a doctor?' How many times have you heard that one already? Whether you've 'just known' since you were knee high to a grasshopper or this has been a recent development, it's the one question that you can guarantee you'll be asked by friends, family, teachers. No other choice for a degree course seems to trigger so much curiosity. Perhaps this is a hangover from the days when doctors were omnipotent and commanding, or perhaps due to a general fascination as to why anyone might want to cut up dead people as part of his or her degree course. Whatever the reason, this constant questioning begins to be a bit wearing after a while, especially if, just like I did, you feel something of a fake because you have no real answer to this apparently vital question.

I did, however, have lots of answers which sounded good, or ones that I thought I was supposed to say. To give you just a few, I wanted 'to help people', 'to apply my scientific knowledge to disease' and to 'serve the community'. Now, I'm not ridiculing these ideals, but if you really went into your medical degree with these in mind then you wouldn't last too long. Surely you would be helping people far more if you went and dug some water mains in Africa rather than spending your time languishing in the library of some veritable medical institution? I would instead suggest that the question 'why do you want to be a doctor?' is unfair, because it assumes personal knowledge of a career that you cannot possibly have yet. For example, no one has ever asked the question of a prospective accountant 'why do you want to be an accountant' and received the answer 'because I like sitting in an office and chasing up tax accounts'.

People choose a career because they are interested in the subject on which it is based. You could study law at university and end up in any manner of jobs; you may only choose to become a solicitor or barrister because what you have studied during your degree interested you enough to spend the rest of your life doing it. The same goes for medicine, but the difference is that, because it costs so much and takes so long to train a doctor, they are interviewing you for your job on your entry to university, rather than at the end.

This is perhaps why the choice seems so important: unlike a degree in biology, you are saying to yourself and the world: 'This is what I am going to be doing for the rest of my life.' At such a tender age I found it impossible to imagine a career at 30 and beyond, so at this stage it is more practical for you to focus on why you want to go to medical school and study medicine, and then consider whether you actually fancy being a doctor at the end of it all.

So why do you want to go to medical school?

At medical school you will study pretty much everything and anything to do with the human body and the human mind. So you'd better like your human biology module at A-level, otherwise you'll be in for a rough ride. Just some of the basic science subjects you will come across during your degree include physiology, anatomy, biochemistry, pharmacology, sociology, psychology, genetics, neuroscience, pathology, histology and immunology, and that's even before you get to the clinical specialties like cardiology, gynaecology, etc. That's a lot of learning.

If the thought of spending days absorbed in books before you even get near a living person sounds quite appealing, and you're quite prepared to spend the next ten years of your life sitting exams, then medicine is clearly the choice for you. For the rest of us, during moments of self-doubt, we can take a step back and consider how truly wonderful it would be to understand how our own bodies work; to understand everything from how our skin protects us from the elements to how our cells turn our Weetabix into a sprint for the bus. We can't escape from ourselves, and you will find that your own body acts as a constant reminder of how little you know and how much you have yet to discover. Which is actually pretty exciting, especially for intelligent, knowledge-seeking people like yourselves.

However, you will be pleased to hear that there is plenty to do at medical school besides study. You may think that your extracurricular activities will stop as soon as you get your place, but, actually, with the new modernising medical careers programme for junior doctors now up and running, it is more important than ever that you get involved in activities and organisations in order to continue your development as a well-rounded individual.

At medical school you will probably find the most diverse range of people in any degree course in the country, all with a single ambition. So, depending on the size of the medical school, you will instantly have up to 450 new best friends! After all the struggle to get to medical school you will find it is a surprisingly supportive and uncompetitive place, and I promise that you will love it. There will certainly be times when you think you can't continue, but they soon pass and they actually serve to make you even more determined.

Why do you think you want a job as a doctor?

Some of you may have decided long ago that medicine was for you and, if so, you deserve congratulations for picking such a great career so early on. Others of you may have personal experience of family members working in medicine. If either of these apply, you'll have realised by now that a career in medicine has a few downsides: the constant exams, the endless lists of knowledge, the late nights, the early mornings, the slow career progression, the constant moving around, the abusive patients… I could go on.

So what makes the very brightest of us want to sacrifice a large proportion of our best years to a job like this? If you think about it, there are a lot of reasons. First, can you think of any other job where you get up each day not having a clue about what you will see, whom you will meet and who or what will come flying at you through the door?

Secondly, you will never get bored because medicine has an incredibly varying routine, limited only by the variety of people in the world. Plus, as you'll never know everything, you can't stagnate: medicine is constantly changing and adapting as new knowledge is added. Thirdly, to the nitty gritty: money. There seems to be some unwritten rule that 'thou shalt not discuss money or working conditions when thou art a prospective medical student'. I don't know why this is. Perhaps it doesn't fit with the self-sacrificing image we think we have to portray in order to get into medical school, but all the same the pay isn't bad.

No one who becomes a doctor is going to get rich quick, but you're not going to be out on the streets either. At present, a newly qualified junior doctor in a 'high intensity post' (that means working your fingers to the bone and doing lots of extra hours) can expect to take home about £30,000. You also have very little potential to be unemployed unless you want to be, and you'll also get an excellent pension. Luckily, the NHS has also got its act together as regards flexible training (that's part-time work in non-NHS speak), so your career won't suffer if you want to have a family (you might not be thinking about that one at the moment, but you'll be glad of it in later years!).

If you weren't convinced before, I'm sure you are now. All that remains for you to do is to get that coveted place at medical school. You are probably aware that a few hurdles lie in your way between now and then, namely, excellent A-level grades, a fantastic personal statement, a resounding score on the BMAT or UKCAT exam and, finally, a jaw-dropping performance at interview. And there's the competition – have a look at Tables 1, 2 and 3 for the 2010 year of application to UK medical schools to see what you're up against.

Table 1 Entry to UK medical schools (2010)

	All applications	All acceptances	Clearing acceptances	Acceptances (per cent)
Men	9,364	3,544	140	37.8
Women	11,574	4,403	193	38
Total	20,938	7,947	333	38

Table 2 Entry to UK dental schools (2010)

	All applications	All acceptances	Clearing acceptances	Acceptances (per cent)
Men	1,485	524	18	35.3
Women	1,862	754	26	40.5
Total	3,347	1,278	44	38.1

Table 3 Entry to UK veterinary schools (2010)

	All applications	All acceptances	Clearing acceptances	Acceptances (per cent)
Men	523	234	20	44.7
Women	1,691	744	118	44
Total	2,214	978	138	44

A glance at these figures shows that the competition is pretty fierce, but it shouldn't put you off. You have as much chance as anyone else and, if you follow the advice and preparation outlined in this book, together with some hard work practising for either the BMAT and/or the UKCAT, you can be fairly confident that you will be as good as they get, if not better.

The next chapter outlines the stages in your application to read medicine in the UK, and the following chapters contain practical advice and tips for each of the stages you will go through. If at any time you feel that this is all a lot of extra work and a bit too stressful in comparison with what your friends are having to go through for their respective degree courses, I would advise returning to this section to remind yourself just why you want to study medicine; suddenly everything will seem much more in proportion.

Chapter 3
Your application to read medicine: step by step

This chapter will help you to:

- plan your application from start to finish;
- organise your time;
- keep your application on track.

The fact you're reading this is perhaps proof that the last chapter did not put you off a career in medicine. As a reward for your commitment, this chapter will help to steer you through all the different parts of your application to medical school, providing you with key dates and deadlines and a suggested timescale for events to help you to keep stress levels down and success levels high. You will find detailed information on each of these stages in the chapters that follow, but you can refer back to this chapter at any time to see how it all slots together.

Those of you who are that way inclined can even tick each stage off as you go along – it may seem a small reward for all the work you are putting in, but keep concentrating on your end goal: to become a doctor. Make sure you involve everyone you can to help with your application: teachers have a wealth of experience and will be delighted to help an enthusiastic student, and your family will provide much needed emotional and moral support during times of stress. Most of all, remember that, while getting into medical school is important, it isn't as important as your health and happiness, so make time for relaxation, friends and the things you enjoy.

Key dates for your diary 2012–2013

2012

May

1   UKCAT online registration opens for all applicants entering medical school in 2013, or deferred entry for 2014
Register online at www.ukcat.ac.uk

July

3   UKCAT exam opens at test centres
Medical school open days

August

16   Publication of A1 results

September

mid-September   UCAS application procedure opens
21   UKCAT registration closes

October

1   Closing date for BMAT exam applications
5   Closing date for UKCAT test sittings
15   Late-entry closing date for BMAT (fee payable)
15   Deadline for UCAS applications for Oxford and Cambridge, and medicine, dentistry and veterinary science or veterinary medicine

November

7   BMAT exam
21   BMAT results published

December

Cambridge University interviews
Oxford University interviews
Oxford University offers/rejections

2013

January

Cambridge University offers/rejections

Cambridge University 'pool'

February

Medical school interviews and offers/rejections

March

31   Deadline for declining or accepting all your offers

May–June

A-level exams

August

Publication of A2 results; Clearing opens

Offers confirmed by universities

September–October

Start medical school!

Preparation timeline

May–August

Practise UKCAT questions before test

Work on personal statement – first and second drafts

Arrange work experience/voluntary work

Choose an area of interest to read around

Attend university open days

Research medical schools

September

Final decision on medical schools and non-medical degree choices

Final draft of personal statement for checking by your teacher

Complete UCAS form and send off

October–November

Start preparation for BMAT exam

Continue work on area of interest

Keep up to date with topical medical news

December–February

Prepare for upcoming interviews

Monitor offers/rejections via UCAS website

March onwards

Continue working for A-level exams

Make decisions regarding acceptances/next steps after rejection

Chapter 4
Preparing to apply to medical school

This chapter will help you to:

- decide if medicine is the right course for you;
- choose the right medical school and course;
- collect evidence for your UCAS personal statement.

While it is never too late to decide to study medicine at university, your application will certainly benefit from an early start. With over 18,000 students competing for a mere 8,000 places at medical school for 2010 entry you can see the competition is fierce. These days, applying to study medicine is a lot tougher than it was even just a few years ago: not only do you have to have the top grades at GCSE and A-level, but you must also achieve a good mark on the UKCAT and/or the BMAT exam. In addition, you must produce a well-rounded personal statement that shows evidence of work experience, a variety of extracurricular activities and a keen interest in scientific matters.

It is, then, perhaps not so surprising that students who have decided early on that they want to apply to medical school always ask me what things they can do to improve their chances. Whether you have yet to sit your GCSE exams or have just started your A-level courses, it's not too early to start preparing your application (as long as you don't neglect your other studies to do it). You will find that a little time invested now will make your life so much easier when the time comes around to apply.

This chapter offers practical tips and advice for preparing all aspects of your application to medical school, along with resources and suggested timeframes to ensure you get the very best result from your application. For those of you with a little less time on your hands, all these tips can be adapted to the time you have available; you might just have to work that bit harder.

Important note: It is also vital to remember that medical schools are not looking for a certain 'type' of person; nor are they looking to produce an army of doctor clones. They want to train students who are intelligent, enthusiastic, committed and driven. So don't feel that you ever have to do something that you don't want to because it's 'needed' for medical school – all these suggestions are just ways of demonstrating to the admissions officers what an ideal candidate for medical school you really are.

Deciding if medicine really is for you

All medical schools want to be sure that they won't be spending five years and a huge amount of government money training you, only for you to leave after a few years, having decided medicine really isn't your cup of tea after all. Similarly, you are going to have to make a choice relatively early on in your life about how you want to spend the rest of it – this isn't something to be taken lightly. Luckily, there are lots of things you can do to research careers in medicine, and you may be surprised to find out about the variety of other careers in the NHS and non-medical professions: there are, after all, lots of other jobs which involve science and healthcare, such as pharmacy, occupational therapy, physiotherapy. It is worth considering whether these alternative careers would suit you better. Even if this research only serves to make you more determined to become a doctor, then they're worth a look, especially as you will have to choose two non-medical school choices on your UCAS application form as 'insurance'.

Exam results

Unfortunately, there's no getting away from it: to study medicine you have to be smart, and you have to prove it by achieving good grades. Before you decide whether you want to be a doctor, it's best to be realistic and look at your chances based on your GCSE grades and your predicted or actual A1 module results. To give you some idea of what you need to achieve, have a look at the requirements below of a typical medical school. You need these results as an absolute minimum; many students will have grades in excess of this. (If you don't quite measure up, either in grades or subjects, don't give up straightaway: have a look at the section on page 22 on access schemes and do some research to see if you could get on a foundation or entry programme to medicine.)

Example requirements
GCSEs
- At least six grade Bs to include chemistry, biology and physics (or Science Dual Award).
- Minimum of grade B in maths and English language.

AS and A2
Biology and chemistry passed at grade A and a third subject (excluding general studies) passed at grade A.

NB: Scottish Highers, International Baccalaureate and the Irish Leaving Certificate are all valid qualifications. Check with your intended medical school for precise requirements.

Finding out about life as a doctor

There is obviously no point in going to medical school if you don't think you would like life as a doctor. It can be quite hard to get an idea of what the daily grind and boring details (such as pay, hours, work schedule) will be like before you actually start the job. There are lots of resources on the NHS careers website (see the useful contacts section on page 22), including job descriptions for doctors and other healthcare professionals, advice on what medical schools are looking for in prospective students, outlines of possible career pathways, and details of pay and working conditions. You can also download the NHS careers publication, *Careers in Medicine*, online. This is well worth a look before you jump headfirst into the application process.

Also worth a look is the website of the British Medical Association (BMA). Although primarily for medical students and doctors, there are lots of useful links and descriptions of characteristics required to succeed in medicine (especially useful for writing your personal statement).

Medicine simulation courses

A number of companies offer courses, often over two or more days, where you can experience what it would be like to be a doctor (see the useful contacts section below). These courses are a mixture of lectures and practical sessions led by doctors and academics, and they offer you the chance to meet other potential medical students and to get a flavour of what it is like to wear surgical scrubs, hang a stethoscope around your neck and talk to patients. For a lot of students who are considering medicine, this is a fun way to spend a couple of days – it's a little like a school trip – and it confirms for most students that this is indeed what they want to do rather than being an off-putting experience. However, the courses tend to be during July and at the University of Nottingham, which may be difficult for some of you to attend.

Students and their parents often ask whether this type of course is worth the expense (courses tend to start at around £200 and can get increasingly pricey if you add in all the extras they offer). If you fancy going and you have the money to spare, then it's probably worth it for the experience. Just be aware that they tend to make a lot of fuss about it being a really great thing to put on your UCAS personal statement and that it will give you an edge in a competitive application process, which isn't correct. As you will see later (see Chapter 6), it isn't what you have done, but what you have learnt from it.

Going on one of these courses is just another piece of evidence that you have considered medicine as a career, but admissions officers recognise the courses for what they are and won't give you any credit for attending one unless you can demonstrate what you have learnt from it. Similarly, don't feel that you will be penalised if you can't make it to one or can't afford to go; you absolutely, definitely, won't be.

University access schemes

Perhaps you're not sure if medicine is for you. You think you don't have the right grades, the right social background; you might even be wondering whether you can afford to go to medical school at all. For a long time, students with these sorts of doubts were put off going to medical school but, over the last few years, many of the schools have been actively recruiting local students who are from non-traditional backgrounds or who have slightly lower grades to attend access, information or workshop events aimed at recruiting the very best students with the greatest potential. Eventually, if these students decide to apply to medical school, there are a variety of entry programmes, ranging from qualifying years to catch-up courses, to enable them to study.

Recruitment for these schemes tends to be at local school level, with activities starting from pre-GCSE onwards, so you should check with your local medical school or look at their website if you think this type of activity might help you.

Useful contacts

Finding out about life as a doctor

- www.nhscareers.nhs.uk – NHS careers website.

- www.bma.org.uk – website of the British Medical Association. Contains lots of information about medical schools and future training pathways.

Medicine simulation courses

- www.medlink-uk.org/index.htm – more information about the Medsim and Medlink courses; aimed at students who have decided on a career as a doctor.

- www.rsm.ac.uk – the Royal Society of Medicine sometimes has lectures and activity days aimed at prospective medical students. Check the website diary regularly for upcoming events or become a member to receive more information.

Deciding where you want to go

Medical schools

There are over 30 medical schools in the UK, and you are able to choose up to four to apply to via your UCAS form, plus two non-medical degree courses. If you start early with considering your university choices, you can really get a feel for which ones you would like to apply for. At an early stage it's best to visit each of the medical school websites; these vary in quality and content but generally have lots of information on required grades, course structures, life as a student, etc. (For ease of reference, I have included a list of all of the medical school websites in the useful contacts section overleaf.)

After you have decided which medical schools take your fancy, you'll probably want to visit them to get a real feel for the place. The easiest way to do this is to attend one of their open days, which are generally held over the summer holidays. You can often attend lectures, speak to students and have tours of the accommodation blocks. It's really important that you choose your medical school based on the 'feel' of it and the course structure, rather than on rumours you have heard about it being 'hard' or 'easy' to get into. The best way to ignore these whisperings is to focus on which schools you want to apply to and then concentrate on making your application as polished as you can.

At this point you may feel that you'd be happy to get in just about anywhere, but five or six years is a long time to spend in a place that you find you can't stand. Also note the difference in course structure. For example, at Oxford and Cambridge you can transfer to another medical school (usually Oxbridge or London) after the first three years, and at St Andrews you can move to Manchester to complete your clinical degree period. Different courses have different advantages and disadvantages, and only you can decide which ones seem right for you.

Graduate entry and foundation courses

Medical schools are now being more flexible in their approach to medical school entry, allowing graduates from other degree disciplines and students who don't have the traditional or necessary qualifications to apply for places through graduate entry (typically four-year programmes) and foundation course schemes (typically an extra year on top of the standard course). The universities offering these options are listed below (see their websites for further details). Bear in mind that competition for entry to these programmes is even fiercer (if that's possible) than that of standard programmes. To succeed, you'll have to show an even greater level of commitment, desire and determination than the rest of us.

Foundation year entry courses
University of Bristol
Cardiff University
University of Dundee
Keele University
King's College London (local applicants only)
University of Manchester
University of Sheffield
University of Southampton

Graduate entry courses
University of Birmingham
University of Bristol

University of Cambridge
Imperial College, London
Keele University
King's College London (University of London)
University of Leicester
University of Liverpool
University of Newcastle upon Tyne
University of Nottingham
Oxford University
Queen Mary, University of London
St George's, University of London
Swansea University
University of Southampton
University of Warwick

Useful contacts

Medical schools

www.medschools.ac.uk – the Council of Heads of Medical Schools website. Contains links to all the UK medical schools and also details of foundation and graduate entry courses.
University of Aberdeen (www.abdn.ac.uk/)
University of Birmingham (www.bham.ac.uk/)
Brighton and Sussex Medical School (www.bsms.ac.uk/)
University of Bristol (www.bris.ac.uk/)
University of Cambridge (www.cam.ac.uk/)
Cardiff University (www.cardiff.ac.uk)
University of Dundee (www.dundee.ac.uk/)
University of East Anglia (www.uea.ac.uk/med)
University of Edinburgh (www.ed.ac.uk/)
University of Glasgow (www.gla.ac.uk/)
Hull York Medical School (www.hyms.ac.uk/)
Imperial College London (University of London) (www3.imperial.ac.uk/)
Keele University (www.keele.ac.uk/)
King's College London (University of London) (www.kcl.ac.uk/)
University of Leeds (www.leeds.ac.uk/)
University of Leicester (www.le.ac.uk)
University of Liverpool (www.liv.ac.uk/Medicine)
University of Manchester (www.manchester.ac.uk/)
University of Newcastle upon Tyne (www.ncl.ac.uk/)
University of Nottingham (www.nottingham.ac.uk/)
Oxford University (www.medsci.ox.ac.uk/)
Peninsula Medical School (www.pms.ac.uk/)
Queen Mary, University of London (www.smd.qmul.ac.uk/)

Queen's University Belfast (www.qub.ac.uk/)
University of St Andrews (www.st-andrews.ac.uk/)
St George's, University of London (www.sgul.ac.uk/)
University of Sheffield (www.shef.ac.uk/)
University of Southampton (www.soton.ac.uk/)
University College London (University of London) (www.ucl.ac.uk/)
University of Warwick (graduate entry programme) (www2.warwick.ac.uk/)

Preparing to write your personal statement

When you read Chapter 6, you'll realise just how important your personal statement is for your application to medicine. There are very definite items that need to go on your personal statement, including evidence of academic commitment to medicine, work experience and extracurricular achievements. Obviously, life is going to be extremely difficult for you when you come to write your personal statement if you haven't actually done anything worth mentioning during your time at school or college.

If you are still a while off applying to university, then you have loads of time to get involved with lots of activities and to read around your subject. If your application deadline is fast approaching, then you need to be organised. Please note that it isn't about doing activities just so you have something to put on your form (although this is infinitely better than lying about non-existent voluntary work) but, rather, a focused way of showing off your talents and suitability for medicine. However, as a general rule, I find that driven people like you tend to be pretty involved in school or college life, so you may only need a little extra help in one or two areas.

Work experience

First, you need to do some sort of work experience in order to demonstrate some knowledge and understanding of the profession you will be training to enter. This is easy if you know someone who works as a doctor but much harder for those of you who don't, especially if you're starting early and are relatively young to be rattling around in a doctor's surgery.

If you have a friend or relative who can help to arrange some work experience for you, think carefully about what you would like to do. Obviously, everyone wants to run down the corridor screaming 'get me the epinephrine' just like in *ER*, but it's not going to happen, and to be honest you'd be better off concentrating on talking to junior doctors, students, even your GP, and finding out what they think of the health service and medicine in general. Please, always remember that people's experiences in medicine vary wildly.

If you don't have a friendly doctor to hand, then your first port of call is your school careers adviser. Often, this person can arrange a placement for you with the minimum of fuss. If that does not work, then contact your local hospital and see if they can accommodate you for any work experience. Many hospital trusts offer programmes which involve either a day shadowing a doctor or as an observer in a specific department. Check the websites of your local NHS trust but note that it's best to inquire very early as these places get snapped up quickly.

Students often ask me whether they will be penalised if they haven't been able to organise any medical work experience, and the answer to that is a resounding 'No'. While it is preferable to try to get some experience, tutors realise the difficulty in arranging it and indeed expect that you will also demonstrate other ways of finding out about medicine, such as talking to doctors or researching career pathways on the internet. In fact, some medical schools, such as the University of Leicester, actually state that medical work experience is not essential, while others state that, if you do say you've done some work experience, you will be asked about it at interview – so you better have something good to say about it.

When arranging work experience, try to think outside the box and realise that there is more to gathering experience than trailing the coat-tails of a harassed doctor all day long. Lots of hospitals require volunteers to befriend and advise patients and their families (see the section on volunteer work below) or even to help deliver the tea. You may even be able to get a paid job in medical records.

You will get a far better insight into the inner workings of hospital life if you spend time there regularly, chatting to patients and staff, rather than sitting in on dull clinics for a couple of days. Your own GP will probably be delighted to let you help out in reception for a couple of days – that will really give you an insight into just how hectic general practice is.

Try to get a variety of experience and explain what you have learnt from it. When I was applying I wrote about how time spent in a GP's surgery made me realise just how crucial teamwork is: if a patient's results get lost in the computer system or are not flagged up by the person filing them, then disasters can happen. When I got to interview I was terrified by everyone else recounting stories of their work experience in which they apparently carried out triple heart bypass with a coat hanger while on their lunch break, but actually they had nothing that was worth saying about their experience.

I know you are all honest people, but make sure you are clued up about what you did. One student I interviewed gave an impressive account of some orthopaedic work experience on his statement and then was unable to tell me anything about any of the patients he had seen, which came across rather badly. Always remember that you are demonstrating an understanding of the profession which you can get in lots of different ways: the more unusual your choice of placement, and the more effort you put into analysing what you learnt from it, the better – you want your application to stand out from the crowd.

Volunteer work

Here's an option that is absolutely free, extremely relevant to your future career, teaches you skills that you can put on your personal statement and actually gives something back to the community. If you find that you don't like working with new people, giving your time up for a good cause or sacrificing some of your social life, then you may realise that medicine isn't for you after all. I feel that there is no better way of demonstrating commitment and dedication to a career in the caring professions than actually getting off your bum and helping others. Plus it can be fun. It really doesn't matter what you do – it doesn't even have to be medical or healthcare related.

Getting involved in a project over the medium to long term (i.e. not just a week before you have to write it on your personal statement) can often show more commitment to being a doctor than strutting about in scrubs for a couple of days. Your first port of call if you want to organise some volunteer work is your college careers adviser or community service organiser (a lot of colleges will have them). If you're still at school this might be a little harder, so there are lots of links in the useful contacts section on page 28 to get you started. If nothing here appeals, try looking in your local newspaper or *Yellow Pages*, or you could even pop down to your local school or hospital to see if they need any help with organising fundraising activities.

My top tip is to pick something you think you can stick with for a good period of time, as then you will get the most out of it. There are so many different activities out there, you should be able to find one that doesn't interfere with your school work or part-time job, etc. While you're involved with your chosen activity, keep a few brief notes on the tasks you do and the skills that you develop, and reflect on why it is enjoyable, what is difficult about it and what parts of it you enjoy least. All these thoughts will be vital when it comes to writing your personal statement in order to show what you have learnt from your experience. Additionally, if you get the chance to attend any training courses (such as manual handling, first aid, etc.) as part of your volunteer work, then jump at the opportunity, and it's always a bonus if you can get some sort of written confirmation or certification that you've done it – it's all extra points for your statement.

Academic commitment

In addition to demonstrating your understanding and commitment to a life in medicine, admissions officers also want to see if you will be interested enough to cope with the continued workload while you are at medical school, and whether you have the inquiring mind and natural scientific curiosity desirable in a doctor. You may think that your A-levels are ample demonstration of your commitment to studying, but unfortunately a lot of the competition has sparkling grades too.

The way that the best students demonstrate their academic enthusiasm and commitment is to read up on an area of science or medicine that interests them. You'll find details in the recommended reading in Chapter 5, but the point here is to start early. The months before your UCAS statement is due in will be filled up with the UKCAT exam, A-level modules and preparation for the BMAT exam, so you won't have that much time for reading then. You can also demonstrate your academic commitment by winning prizes and entering competitions like the Biology and Chemistry Olympiads. In short, make a note of everything you do and read that isn't strictly required for your school or college courses and then it will be easy when you come to write your personal statement.

Extracurricular activities

As if the above requirements weren't proof enough that you are a perfect candidate for medical school, to make your personal statement complete you will have to provide evidence that you are a well-rounded individual with plenty of hobbies, interests and enthusiasm for life. In this way, admissions officers will be able to assess whether you have the ability to maintain an appropriate work–life balance which is necessary for your health, happiness and success while at medical school and beyond. Before you ask, there isn't any one thing that really impresses them, so just make sure you get involved in all aspects of life at school or college.

I realise that doing the subjects required for medical school entry doesn't leave you with that much free time, but anything can be used as evidence, from Duke of Edinburgh Awards or football, to playing a musical instrument or being a member of the film society. Try to put yourself forward for positions of responsibility, such as being a school prefect or president of a society. This will show leadership abilities and impress upon them that you are confident and willing to take on duties.

Useful contacts
Work experience and volunteer work
- www.volunteering.org.uk/IWantToVolunteer – the Volunteering England website. Contains lots of information and addresses for all sorts of volunteering opportunities.
- www.do-it.org.uk – 'volunteering made easy' – and it really is! Choose what type of project you want to get involved in, where you live and what time you have available, and the database will search through thousands of opportunities to give you a job description and contact details. A fantastic resource.
- www.wwv.org.uk – WorldWide Volunteering website. You can find volunteering opportunities in the UK (free) or anywhere around the world (for which you have to pay £10 to use the search engine), so particularly good for gap-year planning.

Chapter 5
Required reading and other tips for success

This chapter will help you to:

- read around your subject and develop your scientific knowledge;
- improve your personal statement;
- prepare for your interview.

This chapter is all about preparing yourself so that you can write the best personal statement and perform as well as possible in your interviews, when you get them. You'll be glad to know that I'm not going to recommend that you read the entire *Oxford Textbook of Medicine*, nor am I going to insist that you know everything about your life beyond medical school. What I do want you to do is to step up from being an A-level student, where you go to classes, get taught stuff, revise and pass exams, and begin to think like the future doctor you want to be. You need to be spending time reading books and articles instead of watching television, and thinking beyond what you need to know for A-level. Now is the time to start questioning, probing and researching.

In this chapter I have included tips and strategies to help to improve your chances of success. Some of these tips were given to me, some of them I have used with past students. All of them seem to work. With a bit of effort you will find that, not only do they make your application a lot easier, but they will also make life a lot less stressful come interview time.

Read around your subject

To be honest, so far you've probably not been stretched too much at school or college. You turn up, work hard, revise for the exams and get the success you deserve. Unfortunately, there are quite a few of you doing that, and not quite so many places at medical school. So you need something else. Time after time I have sat before grade-A students and asked them what they have read recently (especially as they've just told me how passionate they are about medicine) only to be greeted with a blank look or a defensive 'I've been doing my exams'. What would you say if your interview was tomorrow and you got asked that?

Reading around your subjects indicates interest, enthusiasm, an inquiring mind and dedication, and these seem to be exactly the qualities admissions officers are looking for in medical school applicants. It may sound obvious, and even too simple to be true, but so many students just don't find the time and energy to look beyond their A-level books. An extra bonus is that whatever time you invest in reading around your subject will pay dividends when you come to write the academic part of your personal statement (see Chapter 6) and will also help in your preparation for the BMAT and interview.

You are probably wondering right now what it is that I am going to recommend for you to read. There is only one golden rule here: read something that interests you. It may be something from your studies that you want to go into in greater depth, it may be an article on the news about some new cure for cancer that you thought you'd investigate or it may be a popular-science book that grabbed you in the library. Regarding this last option, you'll find below a list of books either that I read when I was at your stage or that I have had recommended to me by previous students who have enjoyed them. Notice that I said 'enjoyed' – the aim here is development, not punishment.

In contrast with your A-level work, you will probably find that it is actually quite refreshing reading about things that you haven't met before and that provide new concepts that are difficult to grasp. Of course, the list below is by no means exhaustive – feel free to read what you like. These are just examples to get you started. If you find you get particularly interested in a certain topic, enlist the help of a teacher or search the internet for further reading. Be sure to make notes on any areas of interest so that you can write about them on your personal statement, but only choose topics you would be confident discussing with a potential interviewer.

Recommended reading

- *The Private Life of the Brain* (Susan Greenfield). A riveting read about what goes on inside your skull and what makes us who we are. If you like this, she's written a few more that are worth a read.

- *The Man Who Mistook his Wife for a Hat and other Clinical Tales* (Oliver Sacks). Fascinating. You will actually enjoy reading this one, and it will give you a whole new insight into the interaction between mind and body.

- *Suburban Shaman: Tales from Medicine's Front Line* (Cecil Helman). Gives you a great insight into what life might be like as a doctor. Also thoroughly amusing at times.

- *The Selfish Gene* (Richard Dawkins). You may have seen him on TV. This man has some interesting theories. Just be sure to take them with a pinch of salt – he is rather controversial and not everyone agrees with him.

- *What We Believe but Cannot Prove: Today's Leading Thinkers on Science in the Age of Certainty* (John Brockman, editor). Quite philosophical in parts, but it will definitely get you thinking and, more importantly, questioning everything you read in the future.

- *Nature via Nurture: Genes, Experience and What Makes Us Human* (Matt Ridley). This book is a great read and will set you up nicely for discussions on whether it is our genes or our lifestyles that contribute to health and disease.

- *Medical London: City of Diseases, City of Cures* (Richard Barnett). Particularly interesting if you are applying to a London university. It describes how illness has shaped London over the past 2,000 years.

Know your medical schools

You may have already decided where you want to apply to read medicine, or you may still be in the process of reading prospectuses and visiting universities. What is critical at this stage is that, once you have decided on your choice of course, you must make sure you know what you're letting yourself in for. For example, it isn't a great idea to let slip at your interview for University A that you much prefer the integrated style of teaching when in fact they pride themselves on the more traditional style of course. Similarly, before you go putting on your personal statement that you are desperate to do an intercalated degree, you had better check that all the medical schools you are applying to offer the chance to do one.

There are over 30 medical schools in the UK that you can apply to, and obviously you aren't going to be extra-knowledgeable about each one, but once you've narrowed the field make sure you request every brochure, leaflet and prospectus you can lay your hands on to find out as much as you can about the course that, hopefully, you will be studying very shortly. Most of the medical schools now have excellent websites that you can browse at your leisure.

When your time comes to go to interview, read up about the course. What attracted you to it? Why study in the area? What do you think are the major health challenges facing the area? (I can promise you, they are very different in central London compared with St Andrews.) What are you looking forward to most about studying at that medical school? Do your research first and it will pay off.

It would be rather nice to get an offer from just one of your choices, but a little flattery goes a long way, and admissions officers who have to sit all day quizzing trembling teenagers will certainly sit up and take notice of someone who's clued up, enthusiastic and thinks that they are working for the best institution in the world. (Note to the wise: you can't fake this type of enthusiasm convincingly, so only apply to places you really want to go to, as opposed to ones where your teacher/mate/postman told you that you'd have a better chance.)

What about your gap year?

I am often asked whether it will affect your application if you decide to have a gap year. The answer is, it depends. Not very helpful advice you may think, but actually the 'depends' bit is dependent on how well you can sell yourself and your plans. On the plus side of having a gap year is that you approach medical school one year older (and hopefully wiser), and that you can bring additional life experience to your studies. On the down side, you are one year further from remembering all that vital stuff you learnt in chemistry, and perhaps you've lost that whole work ethic that was going on while you were at school. So, if you want to have a gap year, you have to prove it's worth the time.

You may be planning to spend your gap year working to earn some cash before university, or you may have plans for travel. Whatever the case, you need to have a clear idea of what it is exactly that you want to do – ideally before your personal statement is submitted and definitely before your interview. It's not good enough to ask for a year out and then think you'll sort it out later. If you are thinking of travelling, it is important to think about where you will go and what you will do during your time. Most importantly, you must set out what you expect to learn from your gap year and how this will help you at medical school.

For example, teaching in an English school in Africa will help you to be independent, will increase your confidence in your verbal and non-verbal communication and will allow you to practise seeking ways around problems. If you say something like this either on your personal statement or in an interview, then they'll probably be waving you off at the quayside with your place on hold until you return. Even if you are working for financial reasons, think about what sort of job you want to get and what you will ideally learn from it.

As long as you can justify the year you will be spending away from medical school, then you won't be penalised. The only point to remember is that, in offering you a deferred place, they are theoretically denying a person in the year below you a place. If you are only an average candidate they may be unwilling to take the gamble that someone better won't come along next year. However, if you are a strong candidate anyway, then they'll be more than happy to accommodate you and your year out.

There is a life after medical school

If you have a doctor in the family or a sibling at medical school, then you may have some idea as to what will happen when you skip out of medical school clutching your hard-earned degree. If not, you may be rather bewildered and worried at the stories that have been doing the rounds about students coming out of medical school with no job to go to, or being unable to find work in the area of their choice.

The truth is that the whole process of recruiting and training junior doctors is undergoing a huge reshuffle, under the title of Modernising Medical Careers (MMC). In short, once you emerge from medical school, you will enter a two-year 'foundation programme' which is equivalent to the old pre-registration house-officer year and the first senior house-officer year. Once these are completed, you can enter specialty training or do general training if you are still not sure what specialty is right for you.

It is well worth having a look at the websites www.mmc.nhs.uk and www.foundationprogramme.nhs.uk and spending some time familiarising yourself with the basics of it all. Also on the website are some excellent case studies of different specialties, which are really useful to clue you up on what you need to do and how long it will all take. Don't worry yourself too much about all the details – you aren't going to get the Spanish Inquisition on it at interview! It is worth knowing a little about it, though, especially as it will directly affect you in the not too distant future.

In short, the best way to prepare yourself for your application to medical school is to treat it like preparing for a job interview. You should research the company's position, its ethos, its strengths and its weaknesses. You should find out about your career pathway and demonstrate that you have the skills and the commitment required to succeed in a competitive arena. Most importantly, come the time of the interview, you need to convince the company (or medical school) that, if they fail to hire you, they will be missing out on the best candidate for the job by far. Think like a professional and, hopefully, you'll hear those wonderful words: 'You're hired!'

Chapter 6
How to write the perfect personal statement

This chapter will help you to:

- understand the purpose of your personal statement;
- plan your personal statement;
- produce a polished, effective personal statement.

It is a fact universally acknowledged that someone who finds it easy to write 700 words in praise of him or herself is probably in need of a good slap. I clearly remember the sheer horror of staring at a blank computer screen and realising that, within a few days, I would have to produce what has probably been the most important document I have ever written in my life. I say this not to scare you but to impress upon you that, just as Rome wasn't built in a day, your personal statement will take a bit longer than your bus journey to school or college on the day of the deadline.

In this chapter we will consider briefly what the point of a personal statement is, what it should include (and what it shouldn't) and, most importantly, how you can make your own personal statement so brilliant that you will be utterly irresistible to medical school admissions officers everywhere.

What is the point of a personal statement?

Your teachers have told you that it's important, your friends are worrying about theirs already and even the UCAS application form online allows you to write and rewrite your statement until you're heartily sick of it. But just why is the statement so important, especially now that you are being assessed in so many other ways, such as the UKCAT and BMAT?

Your personal statement works in two ways. First, the admissions officers who have to trudge through the thousands of applications that land on their desk need something to differentiate Miss A, who has six A grades at A1 and is described by her teachers as 'truly and utterly a wonderful student', from Mr B, who also has six grade As and whose teachers 'couldn't carry on living without him'. Similarly, they want to know if Miss A has actually done anything but study during her years at school, and need to understand the rationale behind Mr B's decision to take a year out.

Secondly, the personal statement gives you a chance to show why you are so ideally suited to a career in medicine rather than law, accountancy or investment banking, and why, if given the chance, you would make more of your place at medical school than the people left behind on the pile.

The critical point is this: if you are applying to medicine you are bright. All of you could, without a doubt, pass your exams at medical school and, with a bit of work, go on to be a competent doctor. But the medical schools don't just want students who are going to pass their exams with the bare minimum of work; nor do they want to produce doctors who are one-dimensional and have vitamin D deficiency from never emerging from the library. The doctors of the future have to have the drive to succeed, the passion to put themselves forward for challenges and the humanity to realise when they have made mistakes and to assess their own limitations. The only real way that admissions officers can assess if you fit these criteria is if you tell them that you do in your personal statement. If you don't put it in, then they'll assume you aren't what they are looking for and pass you by.

Approaching your statement

The first thing to do is to start early. Your statement has to be in to UCAS by the middle of October, and your teachers will probably want to sit on it (or 'check it') for a month before that, which means you probably want to be putting the finishing touches to your statement around the beginning of September (I promise you, it will be such a nice feeling when it's finished). So I would advise starting to write your statement around August. Of course, as this is the summer holidays, there is plenty of preparation that you can do beforehand in order to make the writing whiz by when you have to sit down to do it.

The advice below has resulted from my experience over a number of years helping many students with their statements, and it really seems to work. Whether you are starting to think about your statement a year in advance or are panicking a week before it is due in, following the outline below will enable you to organise your statement in a logical and involving way.

Start with an empty sheet of A4 paper and divide it into three equal sections (see Figure 1). The first section is entitled 'Academic basis of medicine' (this is explained below), the second 'Experience and understanding' and the third 'Skills of a doctor'. Leave a small space at the top and bottom – these will eventually become your introduction and conclusion, which we'll leave to the very last as this is probably the hardest bit.

If you are starting to think about your personal statement early, then this page will be rather empty but, as you get involved with extracurricular activities, complete work experience or volunteer work and read journals and books, remember to jot each example down, and then by the time you come to write your statement it will be a piece of cake.

For the rest of you who have slightly less time, you are going to have to sit down and rack your brains for examples to go in these boxes. At this stage just jot down brief notes and examples; you can work on each section in more detail later.

Figure 1 Approaching your statement

Academic basis of medicine
Experience and understanding (work experience)
Skills of a doctor (extracurricular)

Academic basis of medicine

Medicine is probably unique among the professions in that you will never stop learning until the day you retire. Despite what a lot of consultants might say about themselves, you will never know everything, and what you do know will be constantly proved wrong. Fifty years ago, medical students hadn't even heard of subjects like gene-technology and sociology – today they form a large part of the curriculum. So you can bet that, within your lifetime, you'll be struggling to come to terms with new ideas too.

To cope with these new ideas, the doctors of tomorrow have to be able to demonstrate that they are interested in science, understand the ideals behind evidence-based medicine and actually enjoy studying. This is the section in which you get the chance to demonstrate your thirst for knowledge and your genuine interest in medicine as a science (and you'd better be interested now, because you're sure as anything going to have moments where you are mightily sick of it all during medical school).

A lot of medical schools these days make a big fuss over their 'integrated' courses (problem-based learning, patients from day one and so on). The truth of the matter is that you can't run before you can crawl, and you aren't going to be diagnosing Mrs Jones' haemorrhoids before you know your basic anatomy, biochemistry and pharmacology.

So you had better like studying. They want students who are dedicated enough to choose the library over the bar even when there isn't an exam the next morning.

You have a lot of work on your plate with your A1 and A2 courses, but it's not much of an effort to read around a subject that interests you or to read a 'pop' science book (see Chapter 5). I have lost count of the times I have seen in a statement, 'I regularly read the *New Scientist*'. Even if you do read it, is it really that impressive?

In order to impress, you have to get specific. When I was at your stage, I decided my area of interest would be Alzheimer's disease. I went down to my local library and got out a selection of books, from self-help books for carers of people with the disease to a small science book with theories of how the disease affects the brain. I wrote about this on my personal statement, and in my interview I was asked about it. We had a really interesting discussion about the topic, and I was asked lots of scientific questions about protein structure as a related topic. I think that they must have realised I was interested and motivated enough to get off the sofa and read around a topic of my choice and, although looking back I knew absolutely nothing of the importance of the disease itself, this is what counted and I got the place. The point of this is to show you that there are ways you can prove your academic dedication, rather than just talking about it.

Important note: they don't care particularly which books/articles you read, and they definitely won't be testing you on their contents, so please don't become obsessed about reading lots of important-looking medical textbooks (there's lots of time for you to do that once you're at medical school). Also, never, ever, ever put a book or article on your statement that you are intending to read: you might not get around to it, and you will look like an idiot at interview trying to explain just why exactly you didn't make the time to read it (I have seen this happen).

Read something you are actually interested in so that your enthusiasm will shine through. Perhaps it's something you have been studying at school, like genetics, or perhaps a friend or relative has a disease like diabetes that you wanted to know more about. I'm not that old, but in my day we had to use libraries to find out information. Life is much easier now: pop any old search term into a search engine and you will come up with thousands of sites describing your chosen topic (although stay away from eBay – I doubt you can buy 'everything to do with "Cloning" items' there … try it!).

While you are reading, think about how these 'facts' have been found out – just because it is in a book doesn't mean it's true. If you do this you will start to develop the critical appraisal skills you will use throughout your career. For example, how do we know that HIV causes AIDS? How do they go about developing the new 'wonder-drugs' that are always on the news? You should be able to find a topic out there that interests you; just make sure you read something in addition to your necessary school or college work – it looks so bad if you show no evidence of an interest in the scientific world. Whatever it is, write about it in your statement (see the examples in Box 1), and be ready to talk about it at interview.

Box 1 Reading round: examples

I have been enjoying my A1 biology module on genetics, and I developed a particular interest in cystic fibrosis. During internet searches I came across a number of theories regarding why the disease allele is so prevalent in the Caucasian population, including one which described a possible link between the allele carrier state and resistance against cholera, similar to the possible link between sickle-cell carrier status and malaria resistance which I have already studied. However, I have been unable to find any evidence for this theory, which has taught me that, however appealing an idea may be, it is important to realise that it is only a theory unless proven.

During my voluntary work at a nursing home I realised I knew very little about diseases of mental health. I have since read The Man Who Mistook his Wife for a Hat, Oliver Sacks, which gave me an insight into caring for the residents in the nursing home, and has helped me to deal with my own concerns and feelings about mental health.

After reading a newspaper article about the growing epidemic of obesity in the UK, I have been reading about the different measures being taken to reverse the problem, including public health measures, education and drug treatments. During my research I came across a study in which it suggests that a gene could be missing in people who overeat. However, I found out this was not the case, and in discussions with my teacher I have explored the impact of social and psychological factors involved in diet, which has made me appreciate that disease does not always have a cause-and-effect relationship.

Also in this section you can write about any prizes you have won that demonstrate how much you love science and studying it. For example, you may have won the chemistry prize at school, or received a certificate for taking part in the Biology Olympiad. They may not seem incredibly exciting to you, but if you don't put it in then they can't judge its worth.

Rather than just listing your achievements, try to weave them into a sentence demonstrating your skills so that the award or prize becomes proof that you have such abilities. For example: 'During the last term I have been working hard to improve my laboratory skills, particularly in the areas of planning and precision. This work has been recognised through the award of the ICI Challenge Trophy in Chemistry, which I was delighted to win.'

Once you get started you will probably find that you have quite a few examples, so choose your best ones and try to formulate them into sentences so that the academic basis of medicine statement takes up about one third of your 4,000 available characters. You'll probably find that, at this stage, it is easier to use the computer so that you can play about with words and sentences (but go easy on the thesaurus – it often stands out like a sore thumb when you've been over-using it). At this stage also, don't worry about getting the section into final draft form; this is best done at the end when you bring all the sections together.

Experience and understanding

This is the place to put down all the work experience and voluntary work you have been doing over the past years or months (see Chapter 4 for more detail about this, and for what to do if you've left it all a bit late). Medical schools are looking for students who have demonstrated their commitment to medicine and who understand what the job is about, and the demands that will be placed upon them. I always think that this is a bit of an unfair expectation, as they keep on changing the arrangements for junior doctors so that the NHS when you start may be very different from the one that exists today. But in theory it's a good idea, and as you want to spend the next 10–15 years of your life in training for a profession, you may as well know what you are letting yourself in for.

However, it is this section that probably causes the most anxiety among applicants. Some of you may find it easy to arrange places and so have a wealth of experiences to draw upon when writing your statement. Others of you may not have a friendly orthopaedic surgeon in your back pocket and so are feeling rather ashamed of your two weeks' filing in your local GP's surgery, or voluntary work in the care home down the road. Again, the lesson here is not what you have done, but what you have learnt from it.

If, during your time with the orthopaedic surgeon, you sat yawning while he saw patient after patient, then you haven't really had any insight into a career in medicine. If, however, you went and talked to one of the old ladies who was having a knee replacement and asked her about why she was having it done, and then asked the surgeon why she had to wait so long for it, you probably will have more insight into the health service than most medical students.

A lot of students also want to use this section to describe what sort of job they want to go into, be it general practitioner or cardiologist. My advice here is to proceed with caution: unless you have always desperately wanted to do it and it has been your *raison d'être* for going into medicine, then I would save the space and not bother – everyone changes his or her mind about 20 times during the course of medical school, so it's neither here nor there.

To make life easier for yourself, split this section of your page into three (see Box 2), and fill in the work experience and voluntary work you have done. For each example, write what you did, what you have learnt and why it is important to your future career. Always think whether you would give a place to yourself based on what you are writing. If you wouldn't, then it's probably not convincing enough. Again, always be honest – you'll find you have lots of good examples if you just think about them for a while. I've included a few examples to get you going.

Box 2 Experience and understanding

What I did	What I did or learnt	Why it is important
Two weeks in a GP's surgery	Filing patients' records Observed consultations	Importance of good note-keeping Stresses of general practice How important the non-medical staff at the practice are How computers are so important in the NHS
One year nursing home (once a week)	Chatted to residents Chatted to residents' families Delivered medicines	How to communicate with different sections of society Elderly people are reluctant to complain – need to ask if there are problems Problems with taking lots of different medicines
One week chest unit at local hospital	Attended ward round Sat in on clinic Talked to patients	How medical team works Importance of physio/occupational therapy Patient distress at uncertainty

Once you have done this, transfer your work to the computer to start formulating your examples into prose. So with the final example in Box 2, the week at the chest unit, you could write something similar to that shown in Box 3.

Box 3 Work experience

In order to gain a better appreciation of what life as a junior doctor would be like, I spent a week shadowing various members of the COPD treatment team at Getwellsoon General Hospital. Attending ward rounds allowed me to understand how important good team dynamics are in formulating treatment and management plans, and I was surprised to see that physiotherapy and occupational therapy were more often used in treatment plans than I had previously thought. Talking to patients in the clinic made me realise that uncertainty about diagnoses and worries about serious illness contribute greatly to their anxiety, and I observed how the consultant spent a lot of time talking to his patients to alleviate this.

Anyone reading an example like this would get a real flavour for what you did during your time there (which immediately banishes any doubts that you made it up), and that you learnt something from your experience. Don't be afraid of describing operations you saw or a patient you talked to/followed up. Just be sure to remove his or her details. It all helps to make your statement more vivid and memorable.

Skills of a doctor

The thing that continues to surprise and delight admissions tutors about the students of today is that you seem to have an endless capacity for extracurricular activities: from the Duke of Edinburgh Award to a seat on the student United Nations council, from world chess champions to awards for gymnastics. However, these incredible achievements can literally count for nothing if you neglect to present them in the right way. The admissions tutors don't work on a points system which gives, say, eight points for being world indoor tiddlywinks champion and three points for duck-feeding duties at the local pond-life club. What they are looking for is evidence that you have a good work–life balance and have constantly sought out challenges to develop and stretch yourself.

So, if you take one thing away from this chapter, then take this: for every achievement you describe on your form, you must say 1) what it meant to you; and 2) what you have learnt from it. If you do this I can promise that your statement will far surpass 95 per cent of the other statements in the pile. Have a look at some of the 'before' and 'after' examples in Box 4 to get a feel for what I mean. They may sound cheesy at first read, but just imagine how refreshing it is for an admissions officer who has already seen 500 forms to read one that spells out for him or her exactly how hard you worked for your Duke of Edinburgh Gold award and how achieving it has given you a whole new take on teamwork – not to mention how useful these skills will be once you're at medical school.

Bear in mind that it isn't what you have done that is important, but rather what you have learnt from it and how it has helped you develop as a person now and how this will impact on your suitability to be a medical student and future doctor. A lot of people feel they have to lie or 'stretch the truth' in their statements because they feel a place in the second netball team is inadequate, or painting the scenery in the drama show doesn't demonstrate enough flair. With careful consideration of what you have learnt from each activity plus a well-phrased explanation of why it was important to you that you were involved/achieved your aim, even the most basic of activities becomes an excellent example of your suitability for a career in medicine.

Box 4 Personal achievements: examples

Before

I am working towards my Duke of Edinburgh Gold Award and we are planning to go hiking in the Peak District. This has taught me lots of teamwork skills.

(They think: Everyone's doing Duke of Edinburgh, no proof of achievement, no evidence of teamwork skills.)

After

During my Duke of Edinburgh Silver trip in the Vale of Glamorgan my team ran short of provisions. As a result I have assumed responsibilty for food and water for our upcoming Gold Award Trip to the Peak District. I have developed a spreadsheet which details our precise requirements and I am confident that my organisation will enable the team to perform at its peak during the challenge.

(They think: Not afraid of responsibility, organised, team-player.)

Before

Last summer I went to the student United Nations conference on HIV-AIDS. We attended lots of lectures and I produced a report about the problem of HIV in Africa.

(They think: Very passive, no real show of interest in the subject.)

After

As a delegate at the student United Nations summit on AIDS I produced a report about the problem of HIV in Africa. During my research I had to develop the skills of critical appraisal and became aware of the problems of using second-hand evidence. I was very moved by the scale of the problem in Africa and elsewhere and have since completed a charity run in aid of the Terence Higgins Foundation.

(They think: Wow! Evidence of new skills being learnt and personal involvement in the project.)

Before

In my spare time I play the position of striker in the college second football team. This demonstrates teamwork and also leadership skills as I have to motivate my team to score goals. We won the cup this year; which was a great personal achievement for me.

(They think: Some attempt to show what has been learnt, but no real evidence: rather generic.)

After

My position of striker in the college second team has impressed upon me the importance of teamwork. In the cup final this year we suffered a number of injuries and I decided to substitute myself in order to bring defence players on. Although disappointed not to be playing, it paid off as we narrowly won. The time commitment needed to play has been a challenge with my college work, but has helped me to develop the organisation and flexibility that will be required in my future studies.

(They think: Evidence of teamwork and organisation. I really feel like I know this candidate.)

I have read many personal statements and often the ones that, in theory, should be the most impressive read like a dull list of someone else's achievements (which isn't really ever interesting to anyone but yourself and your proud parents). The statements that are always the most impressive are the ones from students who perhaps haven't had the opportunity or ability to participate in a huge variety of top-notch activities, but have made sure that they have given their all to the ones they have been involved in and learnt a lot as a result. So the next time you're halfway up a mountain or scoring a hockey penalty, think about why you're doing it and what skills you are developing. It's quite hard at first but you'll soon get used to it and it will make for an excellent personal statement.

If you're stuck about what sort of qualities you need to demonstrate, think about what qualities you would want in a doctor who was treating you for a broken leg. You'd want knowledge and skills as standard, but then how about good communication skills, and kindness? You'd also need stamina to treat a waiting room full of patients, but dedication enough to treat each one as if he or she were the first. If you then think of an example when you demonstrated your skills, you'll be well on your way to some great examples and you will make life so much easier for the admissions officers who are looking for these very same attributes.

Introduction and conclusion

I've left this until last as it's often the most difficult part to get right, and now you're over your writer's block it should be a lot easier. A good introduction and conclusion are vital, both to catch and hold the attention and to summarise your statement concisely.

Bad examples of what to write for an introduction include 'since my sister fell over when she was two and knocked her tooth out I knew I wanted to be a doctor', and including random statements out of books. These do make your statement stand out, but only for being stupid. If you have had a long-held ambition to study medicine, then that is fine, but try to think about why you want to do it and then use this as your statement opener. For example, 'For me, a career in medicine will allow me to explore my love of science in an arena full of challenges and surprises' is infinitely better than 'I have always wanted to study medicine as I feel it would be the ideal career for someone who loves science and people' because the first example is much more personal.

The conclusion will reflect this opening introduction and will remind the reader that you have demonstrated the skills and attributes required for a place. This is no place for being shy – we need one final fanfare on the trumpet to clinch the deal. A good example might be: 'Through my extracurricular activities and achievements I feel that I have demonstrated the skills and characteristics necessary for a career in the challenging profession of medicine. I hope to continue my personal and academic development at medical school and throughout my future career.'

Putting your statement together

You have just 4,000 characters to play with on the online 'apply' form for UCAS. But at least you have a character counter on your word-processor, so you should have no problem with this. Only transfer it over to the application form when you're happy to submit it. If you've followed the advice above you probably have too many words to fit on, so go through it and be ruthless: cull anything that doesn't scream 'perfect'. You also need to play around with the sentences so that they don't all start with 'I have', 'I do', etc.

When you have finished with your statement, your teacher will obviously want to see it. Listen to his or her advice, but if you really want to keep something in and you teacher wants you to change it, then stick to your guns. It's your personal statement after all, and too much meddling can take you away from what you want people to see of you.

Important note: if you are applying for other courses other than medicine (for example, your two additional 'insurance courses'), then don't worry about trying to incorporate aptitude for these into your statement. If you're going to go for a medical school place, go for it good and proper, and don't compromise. There will be enough about your love of science and incredible personal achievements in your statement already to satisfy even the most stringent biochemistry or pharmacology degree, and they appreciate and understand the situation that you are put in, so don't worry about it.

Finally, however perfect your statement is it won't look too good with spelling and grammar mistakes, so avail yourself of a spellchecker. But please be aware that it has a habit of changing medical terms into something completely unrecognisable.

After all that work you should have a personal statement to be proud of. Just make sure you save it properly. Save it in at least two separate places, such as a removable drive and your computer area at school or college. Every year computer failures scupper statements a week before due date and you don't need that kind of hassle. As it is very common for interviewers to use a copy of your personal statement as a springboard for discussion at interview, always keep a copy of your statement to revise from the night before. Also make sure you keep all the notes that you have made about your work experience and reading as these will come in very handy to refresh your memory just before your interview.

Chapter 7
Interviews

This chapter will help you to:

- prepare for your medical school interview.

As you prepare for the BMAT and/or UKCAT, don't lose sight of the fact that the reason for the tests is to differentiate between candidates who, on paper, appear to be the same academically. Your scores, together with your UCAS personal statement, form the basis of the decision of whether to invite you for interview. With over 18,000 applications for around 8,000 places on medical courses, and 3,000 applications for around 1,300 dentistry places, a good BMAT or UKCAT score gets your foot in the door, but it is the interview which gets your bum on the university seat.

Will I have an interview?

Most medical schools interview shortlisted candidates, i.e. those who have achieved a good mark on their UKCAT or BMAT and have a high-scoring UCAS form. The criteria for offering an interview vary greatly between universities and it is wise to check the website for the university you are interested in.

Whether a university interviews or not shouldn't make a difference to your application or preparation. If they do interview, you need a good BMAT/UKCAT score to get there, and if they don't interview, your tests scores and UCAS form are all they have to go on, so you also need to score well. My advice would be to choose where you want to go, and start preparing for your interview as early as possible: after all, you're highly likely to be offered one with all the work you are putting in for the tests.

What happens in an interview?

Many interviews take the form of a friendly discussion or chat with a member of the medical school staff and/or a clinical doctor. They'll want to know a bit about you, find out how interested you are in the subject, and see whether you have the type of mind that they could teach easily (i.e. open to new ideas, able to think your way around problems). Hopefully, you followed all of the previous advice regarding extra reading and voluntary work, and so you're going to have plenty to talk about at interview. If not, you can put in a week or so of hard work reading the medical sections of the newspapers and thinking about some answers to ethical problems such as euthanasia, abortion, premature babies, etc. (For more on this, see the section on the BMAT exam.) Then when they ask you 'What have you been reading lately?', you won't sit there dumbstruck or say 'the back of the shampoo bottle'. (Yes, someone really did say this. Luckily it was a mock interview!) Remember that anything on your personal statement is fair game for an interview topic, so make sure that you keep a copy of it to refresh your memory before your interview. They may use it to spark off a conversation with you about your reading or work experience, so I'll repeat my advice that you should only put on items that you are comfortable talking about.

If they ask you about an ethical problem, treat it like an essay and always explore the ideas behind both sides of the debate – this will really impress them and demonstrate your mature and non-judgemental nature. Throwing in a few relevant examples from your reading and topical awareness will also make you appear more committed, so if you know something about a particular topic don't be afraid to share it. Also, while we're on the subject, don't be afraid to disagree with the interviewer if you have a valid reason for doing so. As long as you always back up your argument you'll be fine and they'll probably give you extra respect marks for sticking to your guns.

How to prepare

The best way to prepare for an interview is to practise mock interviews. Ask your biology or chemistry teacher to help you (biology teachers are generally better; chemists have a nasty habit of writing up complex organic compound equations and asking you to draw the product of reduction). Some students find that paying to go on an interview practice day helps them, or even employ an interview coach. If this helps you and you can afford it, great. If not, then you won't be at a disadvantage – have a look online for practice questions (there are loads) and have a go at answering them. You need to cultivate 'pet topics' that you have read around and are interested in that you can weave into the interview. Many interviewers cut to the chase and simply ask you what you want to talk about.

The number one worry that students have is that they don't have a perfect answer to the dreaded question, 'So, young person, why do you want to be a doctor/dentist?' Some people do get asked this question, generally to break the ice, and because interviewers aren't a particularly original bunch. Remember, there is no A* answer: your enthusiasm is more important than a lot of waffle your teacher made you rehearse in advance. Just give your real reasons, and if it doesn't make them feel sick, or run rushing for the straightjacket, then it's perfect.

Finally, I always hear people talking about things the interviewers will do to 'psyche you out', like whistling, or reading a book. If they do happen to do these things (and I doubt they ever would) it's because they're rather rude, as opposed to some dastardly plan to test you. The interviewers really are there to try to find the best in you: they have to fill up their medical school with the best people they can find, so it's in no one's interest if you are so terrified you can hardly speak. The biggest challenge is to become comfortable with talking about yourself. When you find out that you have an interview, practise talking about your interests and your reading to your friends, family, even the old lady at the bus stop – then it won't feel so weird and big-headed when you are sitting in your interview and have to start chatting away.

What to wear

When it comes to choosing your wardrobe for the interview, think conservative. No, you don't have to wear a suit, but you shouldn't go for the 'Saturday-night-on-the-town' look either. Doctors in hospitals no longer wear jackets (for infection control reasons), and some don't even wear ties. So don't feel you have to dress up. Imagine that you are a patient and you were interviewing a prospective doctor who was going to perform some very intimate surgery on you: what sort of image would you like them to portray through their clothes and appearance? If the image doesn't say 'ripped jeans' then they're probably best left at home. It's the same with hair (facial and otherwise): think smart, clean and tidy.

After the interview

When you come out of any exam or interview, bear in mind that your brain is wired up to remind you only of the questions that you got wrong, or the idiotic things that you said in the heat of the moment. Try to forget about these, and think of everything as a learning experience. Try also to avoid the inevitable post-mortem with other candidates: for some bizarre reason they always seem to want to make you feel like you performed terribly, and anecdotally it tends to be the students who had the 'tough' interviews that get the places: if you're not pushed during the interview then the interviewers haven't done their job.

Looking to the future

If you win a place at one of the medical schools of your choice, throw yourself a big party and then make sure you work hard enough to get your A-levels in the bag (it would be silly to throw your place away after all that hard work, but every year it happens). If you haven't been so lucky, then don't despair: if you want to take up a place on your non-medical degree course then make sure you get the required grades: there is always the possibility of getting into medicine via the graduate route after you have completed your degree. Some students decide they are still determined to study medicine and take a year out to reapply. Whatever you decide, make sure you talk over all the options thoroughly with your teachers, parents and careers adviser: you have the rest of your life to either applaud or regret your decision, so it doesn't have to be made quickly.

Part II
Preparing for the UK Clinical Aptitude Test (UKCAT)

This part of the book will help you to:

- understand the purpose and the format of the UK Clinical Aptitude Test (UKCAT);
- understand the format and design of multiple-choice questions;
- understand the different elements of the UKCAT and how to tackle them;
- prepare for the test using appropriate aptitude and reasoning questions.

Introduction

The UK Clinical Aptitude Test (UKCAT) was introduced for use in the selection process by a consortium of UK universities' medical and dental schools. The universities comprising the consortium and the courses requiring applicants to sit the UKCAT are listed in Chapter 1. The test will be used in 2012 for both entry to the universities in 2013 and deferred entry for 2014.

As with the BioMedical Admissions Test (BMAT), or other entry examination requirements, the UKCAT is designed to help universities to make more informed choices among the many highly qualified applicants who apply for medical and dental degree programmes. The test has been designed to assess those skills, traits and behaviours that identify individuals who will be successful in clinical careers.

The UKCAT is an onscreen examination and comprises five subtests: Verbal Reasoning, Quantitative Reasoning, Abstract Reasoning, Decision Analysis and Non-Cognitive Analysis. Each of these subtests will be in a multiple-choice format and timed separately. The overall examination is to be delivered in two hours. (Note that the Non-Cognitive Analysis sub test was withdrawn in 2011 but may be reintroduced at a later date.)

There are two versions of the UKCAT: the standard UKCAT and UKCATSEN (Special Educational Needs). The UKCATSEN is a longer version of the UKCAT intended for candidates who require special arrangements due to a documented medical condition or disability.

According to Pearson VUE, the test designers, 'The test will not contain any curriculum nor any science content; nor can it be revised for. It will focus on exploring the cognitive powers of candidates and other attributes considered to be valuable to health care professionals.'

The types of test being presented by Pearson VUE have been in existence for many decades and are used widely in the selection, assessment and development of staff. None of these commercially available tests claims to have a curriculum content and none can specifically be revised for. However, it has been demonstrated that practising such tests does increase both levels of competence and performance. It also helps to reduce anxiety levels in that applicants are not faced with the unknown.

For those of you who are 'fortunate' enough to be sitting both the UKCAT and BMAT, there is some overlap in the areas being assessed. The BMAT has three sections: Aptitude and Skills, Scientific Knowledge and Application, and a Writing Task. The Aptitude and Skills section includes three separate tests: problem-solving, understanding argument, and data analysis and influence. The problem-solving element contains some numerical-type multiple-choice questions that are of a similar format to those in the UKCAT Quantitative Reasoning subtest. There are also some numerical-type questions within the Scientific Knowledge and Application section of the BMAT. In relation to understanding argument, this may also have some parallels with the UKCAT Verbal Reasoning subtest.

Format and design of multiple-choice questions

This section provides a brief overview of multiple-choice question tests and then examines their format and design and, in particular, the design being suggested for use in the UKCAT.

Which of the following are true of multiple-choice tests and questions?

A   The tests are very simplistic

B   The questions are easy to answer

C   The tests are a poor substitute for real examinations

D   A good guessing strategy will always get you a decent mark

E   None of the above

The answer, of course, is E – none of the above.

Multiple-choice tests have a very good track record in the field of assessment and, particularly, in selection. Multiple-choice questioning is a technique that simply tests the candidates' knowledge and understanding of a particular subject on the date of the test. They make candidates read and think, but not write, about the question set, contrary to the case with essay-type questions.

It is true that there have been a number of long-held criticisms – and myths – about multiple-choice tests. For one, it has been a criticism that they are too simple-minded and trivial. What this observation really means is that it is perfectly obvious to the candidate what he or she has to do. There are no marks for working out what the examiner wants – it's obvious. But this is not the same as saying that the answer is obvious – far from it.

In addition, multiple-choice questions are often referred to by students as being 'multiple-guess' questions, on the basis that the right answer lies in one of the options given and therefore you have a good mathematical chance of happening upon the right answer. Although systematic and even completely random guessing does occur in multiple-choice tests, their effects can be minimised and their use identified by properly constructed, presented and timed tests. The people who design and analyse multiple-choice tests are often just as interested in what wrong answers you give as the right ones. This is because, apart from other things, patterns can be discerned and compared with others taking the same test, and tendencies towards certain answers (e.g. always choosing option B) will stand out.

In short, guessing is easy to spot and unlikely to succeed. Given that the purpose of the UKCAT is to inform the overall decision-making process in selecting you over your fellow applicants (rather than your simply achieving a good score), relying on guesswork is a poor strategy.

Multiple-choice tests are used extensively both in Europe and the USA, from staged tests in schools to university selection and assessment, to some of the most complex and high-stake professional trade qualifications. The strength of these tests is that they can provide fair and objective testing on a huge scale at small cost, in the sense that their administration is standardised and their developers can demonstrate that the results are not going to vary according to the marker – a criticism of essay-type tests. The format and design of the multiple-choice questions used for the UKCAT will undoubtedly follow the general educational model.

The following description of the format and design of multiple-choice questions has been informed by two publications. First, *Assessment and Testing: A Survey of Research* (University of Cambridge Local Examinations Syndicate, 1995). The University of Cambridge Local Examinations Syndicate has been in existence for over 130 years and prepares examinations for over 100 countries. Secondly, *Constructing Written Test Questions for the Basic Clinical Sciences* (second edition, Susan M. Case and David B. Swanson, National Board of Medical Examiners, 1998). The National Board of Medical Examiners, which is based in the USA, uses multiple-choice questions to test in excess of 100,000 medical students each year, including foreign doctors, at numerous sites throughout the world.

In all, multiple-choice testing – properly conducted – is well established, well respected and well used across the professional assessment world.

Multiple-choice questions: 'one best answer' format

There are a number of different formats that can be used for multiple-choice tests but the most common format is that taken from the 'one best answer' family. Generally this is the format used in the UKCAT subtests and is discussed in detail below in relation to each of the four subtests. However, before looking at the specific subtests it is useful first to understand the general structure of the 'one best answer' format.

The 'one best answer' format is also known as 'A-type questions' and it is the most widely used format in multiple-choice tests. This format makes explicit the number of choices to be selected, and it usually consists of a *stem* and a *lead-in question,* followed by a series of *choices,* normally between three and five. To demonstrate this we will use a simple example taken from a typical numerical aptitude test.

Stem

The stem is usually a set of circumstances that can be presented in a number of different ways. The circumstances may be presented in a few simple sentences (as a document, a letter or some form of pictorial display) or may be presented in a longer passage (such as a newspaper article or an extract from a book or periodical). The stem provides all the information for the question that will follow.

A simple numerical aptitude stem could be:

A college had 20,000 students in 1999. Of these students, 8,000 studied a science subject.

Lead-in question

The lead-in question identifies the exact answer the examiner requires from the circumstances provided in the stem. For example, the lead-in question for the stem example given above would be:

What is the approximate ratio of students studying science to the total number of students at the college?

Choices

The choices provided will always consist of **one** correct answer. The remainder are incorrect answers, often referred to as 'distracters'.

For example, typical choices for the stem and lead-in question example given above could be:

A   2:3

B   2:5

C   3:2

D   3:5

Answer and rationale

Answer B is correct: 2:5.

Ratios: rule

A ratio allows one quantity to be compared with another quantity. Any two numbers can be compared by writing them alongside each other, with the numbers separated by a ratio sign (:).

To work out the ratio of students studying science to the total number of students at the college:

Step 1: write the figures separated by the ratio sign with the number being compared first, so here 8,000:20,000.

Step 2: cancel these figures down if possible. Here they can be cancelled to 8:20 by dividing by 1000 and then further cancelled by dividing both numbers by 4 to obtain 2:5.

Step 3: the ratio of students studying science compared with the total number of students at the college is 2:5.

Format of the Verbal Reasoning subtest

This subtest assesses your ability to think logically about written information and to arrive at a reasoned conclusion.

Stem

This stem will consist of reading passages usually taken from books, magazines, periodicals, pamphlets or newspapers.

Lead-in question

For each of the stems, there will be four separate lead-in statements. These statements will relate to the reading passage, and you will be required to determine whether the statement is true or false, or whether you cannot determine if the statement is true or false.

Choices

There will be three choices for each question: True, False or Can't Tell. Again, only **one** of these choices will be the correct answer and the remaining two choices will be incorrect.

Format of the Quantitative Reasoning subtest

This subtest assesses your ability to solve numerical problems. The format of the Quantitative Reasoning subtest is very similar to that described in the example above.

Stem

The stem will consist of tables, charts and/or graphs.

Lead-in question

For each of the stems (i.e. the tables, charts and/or graphs), there will be four separate lead-in questions.

Choices

There will be five choices for each question: A, B, C, D and E. Remember, there is only **one** correct answer and the remaining four choices will be incorrect.

Format of the Abstract Reasoning subtest

This subtest assesses your ability to infer relationships from information by convergent and divergent thinking.

Stem

The stem will consist of a pair of shapes known as 'Set A' and 'Set B'.

Lead-in question

For each pair of Set A and Set B shapes, there will be five 'Test Shapes' which represent five lead-in questions.

Choices

For each of the five Test Shapes there will be three choices: Set A, Set B or Neither Set. Only **one** of the three choices is correct.

Format of the Decision Analysis subtest

This subtest assesses your ability to decipher and make sense of coded information and to make judgements which cannot be based on logical deduction alone.

Stem

In the stem you will be presented with one scenario and a significant amount of information together with terms that become progressively more complex and ambiguous.

Lead-in questions

There will be 26 separate lead-in questions based on the one scenario.

Choices

There will be either four or five choices for each question, A, B, C, D, and/or E. Whereas in the Quantitative Reasoning subtest only **one** answer is correct, in the Decision Analysis subtest there may be **more than one** answer that is correct. This should be clearly indicated in the lead-in question.

How to approach multiple-choice questions

Whatever the purpose or the design of the test, it is worth bearing in mind some general rules to follow when answering multiple-choice questions. Clearly, your score should be higher if you attempt to answer all the questions in the test and avoid wild guessing. However, if you are running out of time you may attempt some 'educated' guesses but, where five options are available, this may prove difficult. If there are questions you are unsure of, you can place a mark against them for reviewing later.

Although it is often repeated at every level of testing and assessment in every walk of life, it is nevertheless worth reiterating – always read the questions carefully. It may help to read them more than once to avoid misreading a critical word(s). With the verbal reasoning and problem-solving tests in the UKCAT, careful reading of the words presented is crucial.

Where all the options, or some of the options, begin with the same word(s), or appear very similar, be sure to mark the correct option.

In relation to the Verbal Reasoning subtest, do not use your own knowledge or experience of the subject matter to influence your answers – even if your knowledge contradicts that of the author. The concept of this subtest is not to test individual prior knowledge – it is to present everyone competing against you with the same opportunity to demonstrate his or her skills and aptitudes. As such your answers should relate directly to:

- your understanding of the passage you have read; and
- the way in which the author has presented it to you, the reader.

Examine each passage to extract the main ideas and avoid making hasty conclusions.

The following four chapters contain details of the four UKCAT subtests and provide practice tests for each. By working through these chapters you will not only familiarise yourself with the format of these tests but will also speed up your reactions and give yourself the confidence to handle successfully the differing styles of questions involved.

Format of the Non-Cognitive Analysis subtest

This subtest identifies the attributes and characteristics of robustness, empathy and integrity that contribute to successful health professional practice.

The format of this subtest differs from the other four as there are no right or wrong answers. The questions will be statements presented in various formats which will require you to indicate how strongly you agree with each statement, how well it describes you or how true it is of you.

Chapter 8
The Verbal Reasoning subtest

This chapter will help you to:

- understand the purpose and the format of verbal reasoning tests;
- prepare for the Verbal Reasoning subtest using general verbal reasoning questions;
- test your knowledge and understanding of verbal reasoning-type questions;
- identify those verbal reasoning skills where development is required.

Introduction

Pearson VUE describes the purpose of this subtest as follows: 'The Verbal Reasoning subtest assesses a candidate's ability to read and think carefully about information presented in passages.'

In the commercial world, the Verbal Reasoning subtest described by Pearson VUE is a classic critical reasoning test. The notion that we all have 'thinking skills' or 'core skills' that should be transferable to all subject areas has attracted a great deal of academic interest. One of these 'core skills' is called 'critical thinking' and the vast number of books on the subject testifies to the interest in – and complexity of – the subject. Critical thinking is fundamentally concerned with the way arguments are structured and produced by whatever media: discussion, debate, a paper, a report, an article or an essay. The following are the generally accepted criteria for critical thinking.

- The ability to differentiate between facts and opinions.
- The ability to examine assumptions.
- Being open-minded as you search for explanations, causes and solutions.
- Being aware of valid or invalid argument forms.
- Staying focused on the whole picture, while examining the specifics.
- Verifying sources.
- Deducing and judging deductions.
- Inducing and judging inductions.
- Making value judgements.
- Defining terms and judging definitions.
- Deciding on actions.

- Being objective.
- A willingness and ability always to look at alternatives.

The above is not meant to be an exhaustive list of all the criteria of critical thinking, but it provides an overview of some of the basic principles that underpin the Verbal Reasoning subtest.

When making selection decisions – whether they are for training, further education or for job appointments – the area of critical thinking/reasoning is deemed to be very important. This is largely because these skills are important in performing the roles themselves, particularly those in management. Graduate/managerial-level aptitude tests of verbal reasoning, which are basically assessing the understanding of words, grammar, spelling, word relationships, etc., may provide an objective assessment of a candidate's verbal ability.

However, these types of test are seen by some to lack face validity (that is, they do not appear to be job related) when used for graduate/managerial roles. People of this level often object to being given 'IQ tests' and prefer an assessment that appears to replicate, to some extent, the content of the job (i.e. critically evaluating reports). It is also believed by some that classic verbal reasoning tests do not provide an indication of an individual's ability to think critically. Therefore psychometrists have developed what are generally called critical reasoning tests, which are similar in format to the UKCAT and are described in the following section.

This chapter provides you with an opportunity to test your understanding and knowledge of the range of questions you are likely to be presented with in this UKCAT subtest. By taking this opportunity, you should be able to identify areas where you may need some development.

Verbal Reasoning subtest

Before attempting the practice questions you should find it beneficial to work through the following example questions. These passages and questions are formatted along the lines used in the UKCAT, using the response options of True, False or Can't Tell. The answers and the rationales for the correct answers follow each question.

The first passage is a relatively short paragraph followed by just one question. Subsequent passages will increase in size and the number of questions will increase to a maximum of four. The final passage, with its four questions, will serve as a 'trial run' prior to attempting the Verbal Reasoning practice subtest. This staged approach should develop your understanding of how this type of reasoning test is structured, and should also develop your confidence and ability when answering the questions.

Passages, response formats and example questions

The passages are normally extracts taken from various books, magazines, periodicals, pamphlets and newspapers. These passages are not a test of knowledge and may not include any medical or scientific-type matters. Each of the passages is intended to convey information or to persuade the reader of a point of view. You must assume that what is stated in each passage is factual and avoid drawing on your own knowledge or experience of any of the topics, which may contradict that of the author. Drawing on this assumption, read the passage carefully and decide whether the statement is True or False, or whether you Can't Tell without more information.

The definitions to be applied to each statement are as follows.

- *True*: this means that the statement is actually made in the passage, that it is implied or follows logically from the information in the passage.

- *False*: this means that the statement directly contradicts a statement made in, implied by or following logically from the passage.

- *Can't Tell*: this means that there is insufficient information in the passage to arrive at a firm conclusion as to whether the statement is true or false.

Example questions

Example passage I: European Convention on Human Rights: Article 10 (Freedom of Expression)

Article 10(2) clearly allows for an individual's freedom of expression to be curtailed under a number of circumstances including the prevention of disorder or crime and the protection of morals. Balancing these competing needs is one area where the European Court of Human Rights has allowed a reasonable 'margin of appreciation'. Nevertheless, any restrictions on an individual's freedom of expression will be narrowly construed and closely scrutinised. Demonstrators may be able to rely on Article 10 as a defence to a charge under the Public Order Act 1986 and hunt saboteurs bound over to keep the peace by magistrates have been able to show their rights have thereby been unjustifiably restricted.

Source: Blackstone's Police Manual. Volume 4. General Police Duties Oxford University Press, 2009. By permission of Oxford University Press.

Example passage I: question 1

Hunt saboteurs who have invoked Article 10 of the Convention have been released from being bound over to keep the peace.

A   True

B   False

C   Can't Tell

Answer: True

In the final sentence, it is stated that hunt saboteurs who have been bound over to keep the peace have shown that their rights have been unjustifiably restricted by this order. The reference at the start of this sentence to the possible use of Article 10 as a defence by demonstrators implies that these hunt saboteurs were able to show the illegality of the binding over order by invoking Article 10. Having successfully shown its illegality, it follows logically that they would have been released from the order. It is therefore true to say that hunt saboteurs who have invoked Article 10 of the Convention have been released from being bound over to keep the peace.

Example passage II: National Minimum Wage

National Minimum Wage (NMW) was 7 years old on 1 April 2006 and since its introduction in 1999 rates have continued to increase each year. When first introduced the minimum wage stood at £3.60 per hour whilst currently, for workers aged 22 and above, this has now risen to £5.05 per hour (£5.35 from 1 October 2006). The rate for workers aged 18–21 and those on a Government approved training scheme has also increased from £3.00 per hour in 1999 to £4.25 (£4.45 from 1 October 2006). And in addition a rate of £3.00 per hour was introduced on 1 October 2004 (£3.30 from 1 October 2006) for workers under 18 who are above compulsory school leaving age.

Source: *HM Revenue and Customs Employer Bulletin*, April 2006, Issue 23.

Example passage II: question 1

Workers aged 21 have not had as big an increase in the minimum wage over the past 7 years as those who are aged 22.

A   True

B   False

C   Can't Tell

Answer: True

In 1999 the minimum wage was £3.60 per hour and now, for workers aged 22, it has risen to £5.05 per hour, an increase of £1.45. For workers aged 18–21 it has risen from £3.00 per hour in 1999 to £4.25 per hour in 2006, an increase of £1.25. Therefore the increase in the minimum wage for those aged 22 is £0.20 more than for those aged 21.

Example passage II: question 2

Since 1 October 1999 the rate for workers aged 16–18 has been £3.00 per hour.

A True

B False

C Can't Tell

Answer: Can't Tell

The passage states that 'a rate of £3.00 per hour was introduced on 1 October 2004 … for workers under 18 who are above compulsory school leaving age'. However, the passage does not tell you what compulsory school leaving age is. Although you may personally know what this is, it is not stated in the passage and therefore you cannot determine the answer without further information. In addition, the passage states the rate introduced in 2004 – without further information, we cannot determine what the rate was for this group before that date.

Example passage III: withdrawal symptoms

The new health Bill, coming into force in summer 2007, provides that all enclosed public spaces and workplaces in England will be smoke-free. The Bill covers virtually all workplaces, including offices, manufacturing plants, schools, shops, restaurants and voluntary workplaces. Vehicles – as enclosed workplaces – will also be caught by the ban. The only exemptions will be workplaces where people also live, such as prisons, oil-rigs, residential care homes, and designated hotel bedrooms. But as in Scotland, the new no-smoking law for England won't say whether organisations should extend the ban to outdoor premises, erect smoking shelters, continue to allow customary smoking breaks, or outlaw smoking altogether. One of the keys to successfully implementing changes to smoking policies is consultation, which gives staff time to assimilate the reasons, benefits and timescales involved. Three months' consultation, followed by three months' notice of policy change would not be unusual, according to lawyers.

Source: 'Withdrawal Symptoms' (Penny Cottee, *People Management*, 4 May 2006). © People Management.

Example passage III: question 1

Staff working at hotels who 'live in' will not be subject to the same no-smoking requirements as the other guests in the hotel.

A   True

B   False

C   Can't Tell

Answer: True

One of the exemptions is workplaces where people also live, and this includes designated hotel bedrooms. It is logical to assume that staff bedrooms are separate within a hotel and therefore would not be subject to any 'smoke free' requirement. In any event, if staff were making use of hotel rooms these could be designated as 'smoking' if necessary.

Example passage III: question 2

The new health Bill requires that organisations provide three months' consultation before implementing the no-smoking policy.

A   True

B   False

C   Can't Tell

Answer: False

The passage does not state that it is a specific requirement of the Bill to provide three months' consultation. It is only according to lawyers and, one assumes, best practice that three months' consultation, followed by three months' notice of policy change, would not be unusual.

Example passage III: question 3

It will be the responsibility of organisations themselves to introduce and enforce the new no-smoking law in the workplace.

A   True

B   False

C   Can't Tell

Answer: Can't Tell

From the tenet of the passage it is logical to assume that the introduction of a smoke-free workplace will be the responsibility of individual organisations. However, it is not as clear cut in relation to the enforcement issue. The Bill may contain both a vicarious liability on the part of the organisation as well as a liability in relation to the individual 'breaking the law' (i.e. smoking in the workplace).

Example passage IV: enabling dyslexics to cope in employment

Sequencing difficulties affect the ability to plan and organise work and express ideas on paper and verbally. Inaccuracies may occur in word processing or writing typically involving letters, or words appearing in the wrong order and words being left out or repeated. Written letters are often the mirror or reverse image of those they should have used, i.e. d for b, p for q, p for b, n for u, m for w. Rotation of numbers and letters through 180 degrees may occur, e.g. 6 to 9, b to q, p to d, n to u, and a to e. Curved characters may be reproduced as similar ones with straight strokes, e.g. u as v, 2 as z, s as 5, and 8 as B. Common tools to help with spelling and grammar problems, such as dictionaries, thesauri and spell checkers, can be difficult for dyslexics to use.

Source: 'Enabling dyslexics to cope in employment' (Patrick Packwood, *Selection and Development Review*, Volume 22, no. 1, 2006). © The British Psychological Society 2006.

Example passage IV: question 1

Dictionaries, thesauri and spell checkers do not help dyslexics with sequencing problems.

A True

B False

C Can't Tell

Answer: False

The passage actually states that 'dictionaries, thesauri and spell checkers can be difficult for dyslexics to use'. It does not say that they do not help dyslexics with sequencing problems – therefore the answer is False.

Example passage IV: question 2

Common problems in relation to letters can be where dyslexics include the letter 'n', which, if written, could actually be a 'u' or even a 'v' dependent on their particular difficulties with sequencing.

A True

B False

C Can't Tell

Answer: Can't Tell

In the passage it states that written letters are often the mirror or reverse image of those they should have used, and provides the example of 'n' for 'u'. The passage also discusses curved characters being reproduced as similar ones with straight strokes, and provides the example of 'u' being written as 'v'. Whether or not an 'n' could be reproduced as a 'v' is not discussed, but it may be that a dyslexic with image and curved character problems could write 'v' from an initial 'n'. More information would be required before a definitive True or False answer could be given.

Example passage IV: question 3

Considering written letters are often the mirror or reverse image of those they should have used, some people with dyslexia may write 'b' for 'd', or 'w' for 'm'.

A True

B False

C Can't Tell

Answer: True

The letters 'b' for 'd' and 'w' for 'm' are still mirror or reverse images and, although these have not been used by the author in his examples, he does use 'd' for 'b' and 'm' for 'w' which can logically be transposed.

Example passage IV: question 4

Dyslexics with sequencing problems may find it difficult to provide a coherent structure when writing an essay or presenting a research paper.

A True

B False

C Can't Tell

Answer: True

The passage specifically states that 'Sequencing difficulties affect the ability to plan and organise work and express ideas on paper and verbally.' It can be assumed, therefore, that dyslexics with sequencing problems would find difficulty in structuring an essay or presenting a research paper.

Verbal Reasoning practice subtest

The Verbal Reasoning subtest is an on-screen test that consists of 44 items associated with 11 reading passages. For each reading passage there are four questions in the form of statements. Three answer options are provided for each statement: True; False; Can't Tell.

Only one of these options is correct. A period of twenty-two minutes is allowed for the subtest, with one minute for instruction and the remaining twenty-one minutes for items.

If the reader wants to simulate 'test conditions', he or she is advised to use rough paper to mark down his or her choice for each of the questions (i.e. True, False or Can't Tell).

The correct answer and rationale to each of the questions are given in the section following the practice subtest.

Passage I: political and social influences on health

The social model of health says that fifty per cent of our health is determined by wider determinants, such as where we live, what our income is relative to other people and what level of education we have. Political and social factors which influence health are not isolated, but interplay in a complex way. For example, research shows that female contraception usage in developed Indian states (e.g. Tamil Nadu) is significantly higher than in less developed states (e.g. Bihar). Both socio-economic status and husband's education are strongly associated with family planning in both states. Religion and caste are associated with family planning in Bihar but not in Tamil Nadu. What explains these differences? It seems that women's education is the key factor: women in states like Tamil Nadu enjoy higher education status and autonomy. On the other hand, women in northern states such as Bihar are strongly subject to traditional conservatism, are predominantly less educated and less likely to work outside their homes. Tamil Nadu has one of the most efficient governance structures in India and the least corrupt state bureaucracy. Bihar, on the other hand, is viewed by many as being misruled.

Source: Health, Behaviour and Society: Clinical Medicine in Context © Jennifer Cleland and Philip Cotton. Learning Matters, 2011.

Passage I: question 1
There is a very complex interaction of factors that contribute to health.

A True

B False

C Can't Tell

Passage I: question 2
In Tamil Nadu female contraception usage is greater than male contraception usage.

A True

B False

C Can't Tell

Passage I: question 3

Unlike women in Tamil Nadu those who live in Bihar are not allowed to work outside their home.

A True

B False

C Can't Tell

Passage I: question 4

States that are misruled, and have inefficient governance structures and corrupt bureaucracies are likely to be poorly associated with family planning.

A True

B False

C Can't Tell

Passage II: the funding debate

Funding of higher education has long been an issue in many countries. This is a contentious matter as only a minority of the population directly participate; in Britain this is approximately 40 per cent. England has seen a significant change in higher education funding in recent years with the introduction of variable tuition fees for students. Previously the state subsidised higher education for many students, depending on their family's financial income. Prior to 2006, tuition fees were set at the same amount for all institutions. Now individual universities can choose how much students can pay for tuition (to attend). Increasingly fierce competition for students had led to some institutions lowering their fees to attract more of them. Welsh students are effectively exempt from top-up fees if they stay in Wales, because they receive a non-means tested grant from the Welsh Government. In Scotland, students have to make no personal contribution to fees except when studying for a second degree or postgraduate award. Alongside tuition fees from students, each institution receives a grant from the respective country's Higher Education Funding Council based on the number of students registered. Those offering professional courses also receive grants from the relevant professional funding bodies (for example, teacher training degrees are funded by the Teacher Development Agency).

Source: *Global Issues and Comparative Education* © Wendy Bignold and Liz Gayton. Learning Matters, 2009.

Passage II: question 5

Students who are seeking a career as a teacher, in any subject, receive government funding if undertaking a teacher training degree programme.

A True

B False

C Can't Tell

Passage II: question 6
Higher education students from lower socio-economic backgrounds pay lower tuition fees than the better off.

A True

B False

C Can't Tell

Passage II: question 7
Generally, students in England pay higher tuition fees than their counterparts in Wales or Scotland.

A True

B False

C Can't Tell

Passage II: question 8
Students undertaking a first degree in Scotland pay no tuition fees as long as they stay in Scotland for the duration of their degree programme.

A True

B False

C Can't Tell

Passage III: can adult learners be confrontational too?

One of the questions our 100 teachers were asked was about the relationship between learners' age and negative behaviour. It is often assumed that it is only the younger, 16–19 (and now perhaps 14–19), age group which presents a challenge to classroom management in post-compulsory education/training. However, one third of the teachers who responded to this question replied that they had experienced or observed difficult or negative behaviour from adult learners (that is, those over 21) as well as from the younger (14–19) age group. Perhaps we should not be surprised by this. The policies and practices which impact on adult learners are much the same as those which affect learners in their teens. And with adult learners, there may be added pressures, of time, of family or financial responsibilities, and of anxieties about returning to education or training. Moreover, for the teacher, the idea of issuing rules to an adult learner, or challenging their behaviour or pulling them up on their language or attitude, may somehow be more complicated than if the learner was a 16 year old. Whether this is right or wrong is not at issue here. What is important in our current context is that they may feel as though challenging behaviour from an adult is more difficult to deal with than challenging behaviour from a young learner, particularly if the adult in question is older than you are.

Source: *Managing Behaviour in the Lifelong Learning Sector* © Susan Wallace. Learning Matters, 2002.

Passage III: question 9
Two thirds of teachers surveyed have not experienced or observed difficult or negative behaviour from learners aged over 21.

A True

B False

C Can't Tell

Passage III: question 10
The behaviour of adult learners can be as challenging as that of learners in their teens.

A True

B False

C Can't Tell

Passage III: question 11
Due to the added pressures experienced by adults, teaching adult learners is far more difficult than teaching learners in their teens.

A True

B False

C Can't Tell

Passage III: question 12
Policies and practices in relation to dealing with the negative behaviour of young learners are different from those for dealing with adult learners' negative behaviour.

A True

B False

C Can't Tell

Passage IV: ethics and mental health law

In historical terms mental health law (and other social legislation, such as the Poor Law) were consistent with teleological ethics. The end justifies the means, and although mental health issues were perceived socially as moral conditions, it was ethically acceptable to segregate the mentally ill from general society for the protection of both. As treatment and understanding of mental health conditions developed, so did the ethics of psychiatric intervention, and whereas teleology remained the dominant school of thought, there was more consideration of the individual as a person, rather than a problem. The development of social welfare, and more humanistic approaches to those who were considered vulnerable, was reinforced by the establishment of the civil rights and user movements. Today's mental health and mental capacity legislation has both teleological and deontological elements. Although a paternalistic theme persists that emphasises protection of the individual and a degree of control which is teleological in nature, the strengthening of service user rights and increased levels of involvement make the distinction that in some situations the means cannot be justified by the end, and an individual's rights are sacrosanct, a view that belongs to the school of deontological ethics.

Source: *Values and Ethics in Mental Health Practice* © Daisy Bogg. Learning Matters, 2010.

Passage IV: question 13
Due to the establishment of the civil rights and user movements the personal freedom of the mentally ill now takes precedence over the previous overarching moral system.

A True

B False

C Can't Tell

Passage IV: question 14
It is ethically acceptable to segregate the mentally ill from general society for the protection of both.

A True

B False

C Can't Tell

Passage IV: question 15
According to teleological ethical theories the rightness of an action is determined by its consequences.

A   True

B   False

C   Can't Tell

Passage IV: question 16

Psychiatrists belong to the school of teleological ethics as opposed to the school of deontological ethics.

A   True

B   False

C   Can't Tell

Passage V: medical sociology – the macro level

At the macro level, medical sociologists study the patterns of disease found in societies and their possible causes. For example, 11.4 million working days were lost in 2008–09 in Britain as a result of 'stress'. Defined as 'the adverse reaction people have to excessive pressure or other types of demand placed on them' (UK Government Health & Safety Executive), stress is a relatively modern disease, unknown in wartime Britain, which nevertheless affects one in six of those in work, and has individual (e.g. poorer physical and mental health) and social consequences (work days lost, loss of productivity) and consequences in terms of healthcare usage (a significant proportion of patient GP visits are about work-related conditions). Stress at work can lead to lowered mental well-being, physical ill health and health-damaging behaviours (e.g. smoking, bad diet). Sociological studies have shown that factors such as lack of power and control in the workplace, job security, low pay, chequered work security (e.g. changing job frequently, multiple redundancies) are associated with work-related stress. Many sociological theories have been developed and applied to explore the relationship between work, stress and ill health ... it is of interest that work stress has been medicalised: people suffering from work stress (often poorly defined) are encouraged to see themselves as ill, in need of the ministrations of experts (e.g. doctors, stress management counsellors, alternative therapists, self-help materials) who are considered to know much more about their problems than they do. However, research suggests that organisational solutions which address the causes of stress such as workload, role clarity and organisational support (primary prevention) are more effective than those targeted at individual coping (secondary prevention) or counselling (tertiary prevention).

Source: Health, Behaviour and Society: Clinical Medicine in Context © Jennifer Cleland and Philip Cotton. Learning Matters, 2011.

Passage V: question 17

Employers are best placed to reduce work-related stress.

A True

B False

C Can't Tell

Passage V: question 18

People in wartime Britain were not subjected to work-related stress.

A True

B False

C Can't Tell

Passage V: question 19

The writer agrees with the medicalisation of work stress and the need to involve the ministration of experts to help in people's recovery.

A True

B False

C Can't Tell

Passage V: question 20

A health-damaging behaviour caused by stress at work might include people drinking excessive alcohol.

A True

B False

C Can't Tell

Passage VI: children at work

Child labour is a subject that still provides fierce debate and discussion, whether it concerns the exploitation of children in the developed world or the employment of children for a newspaper round. These debates are based upon what is harmful to a working child's development and what the nature of intervention should be, given a range of different social and economic circumstances. According to Woodhead (1998), our concern to protect children can easily become distorted by our modern Western sensibilities, leading to inappropriate responses that can make the problems faced by children worse rather than better. White (1996), for example, mentions the case of child workers in garment factories in Bangladesh being thrown out to satisfy consumer pressures for 'child free' products. No attention had been given to the importance of work in the economic lives of these children and their families. The result was that the dismissed children continued to work, but in much more risky conditions in the informal and street economy. They had reduced earnings, worse nutrition and poorer health compared with the minority who had retained employment. The children themselves believed that light factory work combined with attending school for two or three hours a week was the best solution to their poverty. A new scheme was eventually introduced in which employers linked re-employment with schooling and future employment.

Source: *Early Childhood Studies* © Jenny Willan, Rod Parker-Rees and Jan Savage. Learning Matters, 2004.

Passage VI: question 21
Employers of children in garment factories in Bangladesh provide education for the children and offer employment when they are post school age.

A   True

B   False

C   Can't Tell

Passage VI: question 22
There is concern about the exploitation of children across both developed and developing countries.

A   True

B   False

C   Can't Tell

Passage VI: question 23
Consumer pressure for 'child free' products has been harmful to the well-being of children working in Asian garment factories.

A   True

B   False

C   Can't Tell

Passage VI: question 24
Families with children working in the informal economy were better off economically than families with children working in the formal economy.

A   True

B   False

C   Can't Tell

Passage VII: poverty and education

Even by 2002 three out of every ten Romanians were poor; one out of ten, extremely poor. At the same time, there is a strong positive association between economic growth and poverty reduction. Several variables predict poverty, but multivariate regressions show that the key correlate of poverty is education, with Roma ethnicity and being unemployed second and third in importance, respectively. Rural residents have more than double the probability of being poor than urban residents and rural areas account for 67 per cent of total poverty. (Berryman et al., 2007)

Source: *Primary practices and curriculum comparisons,* © Jackie Barbera and Deirdre Hewitt, *Global Issues and Comparative Education.* Learning Matters, 2009.

Passage VII: question 25
In Romania ethnicity tends to predict a person's socio-economic standing in society.

A   True

B   False

C   Can't Tell

Passage VII: question 26
Over 40 per cent of urban residents in Romania live in poverty.

A   True

B   False

C   Can't Tell

Passage VII: question 27
The majority of the population residing in Romania's urban areas are not of Roma ethnicity.

A   True

B   False

C   Can't Tell

Passage VII: question 28
Improving education in Romania is likely to help to reduce poverty in rural areas.

A   True

B   False

C   Can't Tell

Passage VIII: education for citizenship

The 'Crick' Report, *Education for Citizenship and the Teaching of Democracy in Schools*, was commissioned as a governmental response to fears of social disengagement and civic apathy among young people in Britain and as an antidote to the perceived corrosive influence of much of contemporary culture. In 2002, citizenship education became a statutory requirement of all English secondary schools. It included three distinct strands: *moral and social responsibility*, *community involvement* and *political literacy*. In 2007 it was recommended that a fourth strand be developed, *Identity and diversity: living together in the UK*, intended specifically to address additional and growing concerns that British society was insufficiently 'cohesive' and did not adequately consider itself a united community.

Source: Learning in Contemporary Culture © Will Curtis and Alice Pettigrew. Learning Matters, 2009.

Passage VIII: question 29

Issues concerning race and equality are not contained in the citizenship curriculum.

A True

B False

C Can't Tell

Passage VIII: question 30

The curriculum for secondary schools in Wales, Scotland and Northern Ireland does not include citizenship as a statutory requirement.

A True

B False

C Can't Tell

Passage VIII: question 31

Citizenship has been included as part of the curriculum in England partly because of young people's lack of interest in their local communities.

A True

B False

C Can't Tell

Passage VIII: question 32

Britain has become a pluralist society where small groups maintain their unique cultural identities to the detriment of community cohesion.

A True

B False

C Can't Tell

Passage IX: origin of knowledge

The origin and acquisition of knowledge in humans has been a matter of intense philosophical debate which can be traced back at least to Plato. Historically, views have tended to fall within one of three main camps: nativists considered all individuals to be born with the knowledge they needed and that anything else was acquired by some innate or inherited characteristic; empiricists considered all individuals to acquire knowledge out of experience; and rationalists considered all individuals to acquire knowledge by engaging in reasoning. Today, individuals are considered to be born at least partly 'hard-wired' with an architecture of the mind which facilitates cognition, rather than with a mind full of knowledge *per se*. Understanding that architecture is fundamental to understanding how we learn.

Source: The mystery of learning © John Sharp and Barbara Murphy, *Education Studies: An issues-based approach*, Second edition. Learning Matters, 2009.

Passage IX: question 33
Historically it was thought that humans acquire knowledge genetically, through experience, or by the use of reasoning.

A True

B False

C Can't Tell

Passage IX: question 34
Empiricists believed that humans only attained knowledge through experience and not through education.

A True

B False

C Can't Tell

Passage IX: question 35
Nativists believed that knowledge was not acquired from others or by training or education.

A True

B False

C Can't Tell

Passage IX: question 36

Understanding the mental processes inherited by children will improve the level of educational attainment.

A True

B False

C Can't Tell

Passage X: 'tweenies' and 'tweenagers'

The terms 'tweenies' and 'tweenagers' have emerged within the last ten years to explain recent cultural changes in pre-teenage childhood cohort. Originally coined to term a marketing demographic, 'tweenagers' are 8 to 12 year-old children who appear to exhibit characteristics of teenagers more than those of children. The *branding* and *commercial appropriation* (Russell and Tyler, 2002) of childhood, and especially female childhood, has resulted in disturbing trends ... The key characteristics of an emergent 'tweenager' age cohort include: *educational pressures*, especially national tests; '*pester power*', parents with less time to spend with their children and increasing numbers of divorces might be more likely to consent to demands; *marketing and consumption patterns*, such as mobile phones, accessories, jewellery, make up; *celebrity culture*, infantilisation of celebrity and especially young females; *peer pressure*, to look a certain way, to grow up fast, to try drugs and alcohol.

Source: *Learning in Contemporary Culture* © Will Curtis and Alice Pettigrew. Learning Matters, 2009.

Passage X: question 37

Young people are confronted with stresses and demands that they do not have the experience to cope with.

A True

B False

C Can't Tell

Passage X: question 38

Generally, 'tweenagers' have more commodities targeted at them and more power than this age group will have ever experienced before.

A True

B False

C Can't Tell

Passage X: question 39
Females are more likely to exhibit the characteristics of a 'tweenager' than males.

A True

B False

C Can't Tell

Passage X: question 40
Children aged 8 to 12 have only exhibited the characteristics of 'tweenagers' over the past ten years.

A True

B False

C Can't Tell

Passage XI: *global studies*

Every country in the world, with the exceptions of the USA and Somalia, is a signatory to the United Nations Convention on the Rights of the Child (UNCRC) ... The convention contains 54 articles (points) in which children's rights are recognised and obligations placed on states (governments) to recognise these rights in practice ... The definition of a child under the convention is anyone under the age of 18 ... In their most recent report to the UN inspectors, the four Children's Commissioners for England, Scotland, Wales and Northern Ireland identified the following infringements of the UNCRC which they say deny hope and opportunity to many of Britain's 14 million children and adolescents: *a punitive juvenile justice system; public attitudes that demonise teenagers; lack of protection against physical punishment in the home and one of the highest levels of child poverty in Europe* (Carvel 2008).

Source: *Education and Social Care: friends or foes?* © Sue K Flowers, *Global Issues and Comparative Education.* Learning Matters, 2009.

Passage XI: question 41
Students in full-time education in universities or colleges are not protected by the UNCRC.

A True

B False

C Can't Tell

Passage XI: question 42

The youth courts in Britain are more concerned with punishing children rather than rehabilitating them.

A True

B False

C Can't Tell

Passage XI: question 43

More children in Britain are physically abused by a parent or guardian than any other UNCRC signatory.

A True

B False

C Can't Tell

Passage XI: question 44

There is a public perception in Britain today that adolescents are malevolent and evil.

A True

B False

C Can't Tell

Verbal Reasoning practice subtest: answers

Question number	Correct response	Question number	Correct response
1	A – True	23	A – True
2	C – Can't Tell	24	B – False
3	B – False	25	A – True
4	C – Can't Tell	26	B – False
5	A – True	27	C – Can't Tell
6	C – Can't Tell	28	A – True
7	A – True	29	B – False
8	C – Can't Tell	30	C – Can't Tell
9	C – Can't Tell	31	A – True
10	A – True	32	C – Can't Tell
11	C – Can't Tell	33	A – True
12	B – False	34	B – False
13	B – False	35	A – True
14	C – Can't Tell	36	C – Can't Tell
15	A – True	37	C – Can't Tell
16	C – Can't Tell	38	A – True
17	A – True	39	A – True
18	C – Can't Tell	40	B – False
19	B – False	41	B – False
20	C – Can't Tell	42	C – Can't Tell
21	C – Can't Tell	43	C – Can't Tell
22	A – True	44	A – True

Verbal Reasoning practice subtest: explanation of answers

Passage I: political and social influences on health

Passage I: question 1

There is a very complex interaction of factors that contribute to health.

Answer: True

The answer to this question can be found in the first two sentences of the passage and specifically, '... health is determined by wider determinants, such as where we live, what our income is relative to other people and what level of education we have. Political and social factors which influence health are not isolated, but interplay in a complex way'. From this extract it can be asserted that there is a very complex interaction of factors that contribute to health.

Passage I: question 2

In Tamil Nadu female contraception usage is greater than male contraception usage.

Answer: Can't Tell

Although the passage directly states, '... research shows that female contraception usage in developed Indian states (e.g. Tamil Nadu) is significantly higher than in less developed states ...' it provides no comparison of male contraception usage. In the reference to male contraception in the passage, 'Both socio-economic status and husband's education are strongly associated with family planning in both states' there is no indication as to the extent of male contraception usage.

Passage I: question 3

Unlike women in Tamil Nadu those who live in the Bihar are not allowed to work outside their home.

Answer: False

The passage states, '... women in northern states such as Bihar are strongly subject to traditional conservatism, are predominantly less educated and less likely to work outside their homes.' It does not say that they may not work outside their homes, only that they are 'less likely' to do so.

Passage I: question 4

States that are misruled, have inefficient governance structures and corrupt bureaucracies are likely to be poorly associated with family planning.

Answer: Can't Tell

Although, from the information contained in the passage, this statement might apply to the state of Bihar, it could not be accepted as a general rule without further research and relevant information.

Passage II: the funding debate

Passage II: question 5

Students who are seeking a career as a teacher, in any subject, receive government funding if undertaking a teacher training degree programme.

Answer: True

The passage quite clearly states that students undertaking '... professional courses also receive grants from the relevant professional funding bodies, (for example, teacher training degrees are funded by the Teacher Development Agency).' The 'subject' the student selects is irrelevant to the answer.

Passage II: question 6

Higher education students from lower socio-economic backgrounds pay lower tuition fees than the better off.

Answer: Can't Tell

In reality, students from lower socio-economic backgrounds may receive financial support and pay lower tuition fees than the better off – certainly, the passage states that 'Previously the state subsidised higher education for many students, depending on their family's financial income'. However, there is no information in the passage about the current situation with regard to subsidies or means-tested grants for students, and further details would be required.

Passage II: question 7

Generally, students in England pay higher tuition fees than their counterparts in Wales or Scotland.

Answer: True

The passage states that 'Welsh students are effectively exempt from top-up fees if they stay in Wales, because they receive a non-means tested grant from the Welsh Government', and 'In Scotland, students have to make no personal contribution to fees except when studying for a second degree or postgraduate award.' Generally, in England students have to pay tuition fees even though these may vary between educational institutions.

Passage II: question 8

Students undertaking a first degree in Scotland pay no tuition fees as long as they stay in Scotland for the duration of their degree programme.

Answer: Can't Tell

The passage states that 'In Scotland, students have to make no personal contribution to fees except when studying for a second degree or postgraduate award.' It might be assumed that, similarly to Welsh students, Scottish students pay no personal contribution to fees for first degrees if they stay in Scotland. However, this is not stated categorically. Also, it is not made clear whether the 'no personal contribution' applies only to Scottish students or also to students from other countries studying in Scotland. Further information would be required to determine a True or False answer.

Passage III: can adult learners be confrontational too?

Passage III: question 9

Two thirds of teachers surveyed have not experienced or observed difficult or negative behaviour from learners aged over 21.

Answer: Can't Tell

The passage states that of 100 teachers that were asked about the relationship between learners' age and negative behaviour, one third of the teachers who responded to this question replied that they had experienced or observed difficult or negative behaviour from adult learners (that is, those over 21). At first glance it might be assumed therefore that the remaining two thirds of teachers had not experienced negative behaviour in adult learners. However, the passage actually states 'one third of the teachers who responded to this question' which might suggest that not all of the 100 teachers actually responded to the question. Consequently, further details would be required to confirm this or otherwise before a definitive answer to this statement could be made.

Passage III: question 10

The behaviour of adult learners can be as challenging as that of learners in their teens.

Answer: True

This statement is True as the passage states, '... one third of the teachers ... experienced or observed difficult or negative behaviour from adult learners (that is, those over 21) as well as from the younger (14–19) age group.'

Passage III: question 11

Due to the added pressures experienced by adults, teaching adult learners is far more difficult than teaching learners in their teens.

Answer: Can't Tell

The passage says that difficult or negative behaviour is displayed by both adults and young learners and goes on to identify some pressures experienced by adult learners (e.g. time, family, financial responsibilities). Pressures experienced by young learners are not mentioned. However, we cannot be sure that problematic adult behaviour is directly related to the added pressures described – the passage suggests these may be a factor affecting the behaviour of adult learners, but no evidence for this conjecture is given. The passage does say that '… for the teacher, the idea of issuing rules to an adult learner, or challenging their behaviour or pulling them up on their language or attitude, may somehow be more complicated than if the learner was a 16 year old.' It goes on to say that the teacher '… may feel as though challenging behaviour from an adult is more difficult to deal with than challenging behaviour from a young learner, particularly if the adult in question is older than you are.' So we can assume that some teachers, at least, might feel that teaching adults is more difficult than teaching learners in their teens, but we cannot assume, without further information, that such teaching is 'far more difficult', and so the answer must be Can't Tell.

Passage III: question 12

Policies and practices in relation to dealing with the negative behaviour of young learners are different from those for dealing with adult learners' negative behaviour.

Answer: False

The passage clearly states that 'The policies and practices which impact on adult learners are much the same as those which affect learners in their teens.' In any case, the passage does not state that these policies and practices relate to dealing with negative behaviour. Therefore the statement is false.

Passage IV: ethics and mental health law

Passage IV: question 13

Due to the establishment of the civil rights and user movements the personal freedom of the mentally ill now takes precedence over the previous overarching moral system.

Answer: False

Although the civil rights and user movements helped in the development of social welfare and more humanistic approaches to the mentally ill, the passage actually states, '… a paternalistic theme persists that emphasises protection of the individual and a degree of control which is teleological in nature …'

Passage IV: question 14

It is ethically acceptable to segregate the mentally ill from general society for the protection of both.

Answer: Can't Tell

This statement essentially repeats the second sentence of the passage, i.e. '... it was ethically acceptable to segregate the mentally ill from general society for the protection of both.' The passage statement is in the past tense (was) whereas the question statement is in the present tense and may lead to a False answer being considered. There may well be occasions where a mentally ill person may be deemed such a danger to him/herself or others that it is morally correct for that person to be segregated from general society, and this may lead to a True answer being considered. However, this is not contained within the passage and the answer must therefore be Can't Tell as the statement itself is unclear and would need further clarification for a False or True answer to be given.

Passage IV: question 15

According to teleological ethical theories the rightness of an action is determined by its consequences.

Answer: True

Teleology is defined at the beginning of the passage, 'The end justifies the means, and although mental health issues were perceived socially as moral conditions, it was ethically acceptable to segregate the mentally ill from general society for the protection of both.' It advocated paternalistic policies with an overarching moral system overriding personal freedom in some circumstances.

Passage IV: question 16

Psychiatrists belong to the school of teleological ethics as opposed to the school of deontological ethics.

Answer: Can't Tell

The reference to psychiatry is contained in the fourth sentence of the passage, 'As treatment and understanding of mental health conditions developed, so did the ethics of psychiatric intervention, and whereas teleology remained the dominant school of thought, there was more consideration of the individual as a person, rather than a problem.' From this reference it is not possible to determine whether psychiatrists belonged to the school of teleological ethics or deontological ethics, or both.

Passage V: medical sociology – the macro level

Passage V: question 17
Employers are best placed to reduce work-related stress.

Answer: True

The passage states, 'However, research suggests that organisational solutions which address the causes of stress such as workload, role clarity and organisational support (primary prevention) are more effective than those targeted at individual coping (secondary prevention) or counselling (tertiary prevention).' It therefore follows that employers appear to hold the key to reducing stress in the workplace.

Passage V: question 18
People in wartime Britain were not subjected to work-related stress.

Answer: Can't Tell

The passage states, '… stress is a relatively modern disease, unknown in wartime Britain …' Although not mentioned in the passage there is little doubt that work-related stress has been with us since time immemorial or at least since employment began. However, more information would have been required in the passage to make a definitive statement.

Passage V: question 19
The writer agrees with the medicalisation of work stress and the need to involve the ministration of experts to help in people's recovery.

Answer: False

This answer is supported by the passage which states, '… it is of interest that work stress has been medicalised: people suffering from work stress (often poorly defined) are encouraged to see themselves as ill, in need of the ministrations of experts (e.g. doctors, stress management counsellors, alternative therapists, self-help materials) who are considered to know much more about their problems than they do.' This displays a degree of cynicism by the writer who appears to question the medicalisation of work stress and the use of experts.

Passage V: question 20
A health-damaging behaviour caused by stress at work might include people dinking excessive alcohol.

Answer: Can't Tell

The passage states, 'Stress at work can lead to lowered mental well-being, physical ill health and health-damaging behaviours (e.g. smoking, bad diet).' Although it might be assumed that 'drinking excessive alcohol' is undoubtedly a health-damaging behaviour that may be caused by stress at work it does not specifically state this in the passage. More information would be required to confirm this.

Passage VI: children at work

Passage VI: question 21

Employers of children in garment factories in Bangladesh provide education for the children and offer employment when they are post school age.

Answer: Can't Tell

Although the passage states that 'A new scheme was eventually introduced in which employers linked re-employment with schooling and future employment', it is not clear that the employers actually *provide* education and future employment. The 'link' could be less direct than this. It is also not clear whether or not this scheme applies to all garment factories in Bangladesh. Further information would be required, so the answer must be Can't Tell.

Passage VI: question 22

There is concern about the exploitation of children across both developed and developing countries.

Answer: True

The passage states explicitly that there is 'fierce debate and discussion, whether it concerns the exploitation of children in the developed world or the employment of children for a newspaper round.'

Passage VI: question 23

Consumer pressure for 'child free' products has been harmful to the well-being of children working in Asian garment factories.

Answer: True

The passage clearly states '… child workers in garment factories in Bangladesh being thrown out to satisfy consumer pressures for 'child free' products. No attention had been given to the importance of work in the economic lives of these children and their families. The result was that the dismissed children continued to work, but in much more risky conditions in the informal and street economy. They had reduced earnings, worse nutrition and poorer health compared with the minority who had retained employment.'

Passage VI: question 24

Families with children working in the informal economy were better off economically than families with children working in the formal economy.

Answer: False

The passage states that 'the dismissed children continued to work, but in much more risky conditions in the informal and street economy. They had reduced earnings … compared with the minority who had retained employment.' In this context the 'formal' economy relates to those children employed in garment factories.

Passage VII: poverty and education

Passage VII: question 25

In Romania ethnicity tends to predict a person's socio-economic standing in society.

Answer: True

The passage clearly states that Roma ethnicity is the second most important factor in predicting poverty.

Passage VII: question 26

Over 40 per cent of urban residents in Romania live in poverty.

Answer: False

The passage states 'rural areas account for 67 per cent of total poverty'. Therefore urban areas must account for 33 percent of total poverty and not 'over 40 per cent' as posed in the statement.

Passage VII: question 27

The majority of the population residing in Romania's urban areas are not of Roma ethnicity.

Answer: Can't Tell

No information is provided in the passage in relation to the ethnic distribution of the population in Romania.

Passage VII: question 28

Improving education in Romania is likely to help to reduce poverty in rural areas.

Answer: True

The passage states 'Several variables predict poverty, but multivariate regressions show that the key correlate of poverty is education' and therefore education is likely to help to reduce poverty.

Passage VIII: education for citizenship

Passage VIII: question 29

Issues concerning race and equality are not contained in the citizenship curriculum.

Answer: False

The passage states 'In 2007 it was recommended that a fourth strand be developed, *Identity and diversity: living together in the UK.*' From this it can be assumed that 'race' is part of the curriculum. Equality may also stem from this addition to the curriculum but would certainly be included within the strand *moral and social responsibility.*

Passage VIII: question 30

The curriculum for secondary schools in Wales, Scotland and Northern Ireland does not include citizenship as a statutory requirement.

Answer: Can't Tell

The 'Crick' Report dealt with issues of citizenship across Britain and the development of a fourth strand to the curriculum specifically mentions the UK and British society. However, the passage states 'In 2002, citizenship education became a statutory requirement of all English secondary schools.' There is no mention of it being a statutory requirement in Wales, Scotland and Northern Ireland.

Passage VIII: question 31

Citizenship has been included as part of the curriculum in England partly because of young people's disinterest in their local communities.

Answer: True

The passage refers to concerns about people's disinterest in their communities on three occasions. Specifically in relation to young people the passage states 'fears of social disengagement and civic apathy among young people in Britain'. One of the three distinct strands is *community involvement* and the fourth strand refers to *Identity and diversity: living together in the UK.*

Passage VIII: question 32

Britain has become a pluralist society where small groups maintain their unique cultural identities to the detriment of community cohesion.

Answer: Can't Tell

Although this may in part be true, the passage does not contain sufficient information to justify this response. It does not mention pluralism as a cause for the breakdown in community involvement.

Passage IX: origin of knowledge

Passage IX: question 33

Historically it was thought that humans acquire knowledge genetically, through experience, or by the use of reasoning.

Answer: True

Nativists believe humans acquire knowledge genetically: 'all individuals to be born with the knowledge they needed and that anything else was acquired by some innate or inherited characteristic; empiricists considered all individuals to acquire knowledge out of experience, and rationalists considered all individuals to acquire knowledge by engaging in reasoning.'

Passage IX: question 34

Empiricists believed that humans only attained knowledge through experience and not through education.

Answer: False

The passage states 'empiricists considered all individuals to acquire knowledge out of experience'. It does not mention 'education' specifically but it can be defined as any act or experience that has a formative effect on the individual.

Passage IX: question 35

Nativists believed that knowledge was not acquired from others or by training or education.

Answer: True

The passage states 'nativists considered all individuals to be born with the knowledge they needed and that anything else was acquired by some innate or inherited characteristic'. In this sense nativists did not believe knowledge to be acquired by training or education.

Passage IX: question 36

Understanding the mental processes inherited by children will improve the level of educational attainment.

Answer: Can't Tell

The passage states 'Today, individuals are considered to be born at least partly "hard-wired" with an architecture of the mind which facilitates cognition, rather than with a mind full of knowledge *per se*. Understanding that architecture is fundamental to understanding how we learn.' Although understanding how we learn may improve the level of educational attainment, this is not mentioned in the passage and further information would be required.

Passage X: 'tweenies' and 'tweenagers'

Passage X: question 37

Young people are confronted with stresses and demands that they do not have the experience to cope with.

Answer: Can't Tell

This is a very generalised statement and although the passage clearly indicates the pressures to which young people are exposed, and although it may be the case, the passage does not elicit any information on their abilities to cope with these pressures.

Passage X: question 38

Generally, 'tweenagers' have more commodities targeted at them and more power than this age group will have ever experienced before.

Answer: True

In relation to commodities the passage clearly states 'marketing and consumption patterns, such as mobile phones, accessories, jewellery, make up', etc. In relation to 'more power' the passage states 'parents with less time to spend with their children and increasing numbers of divorces might be more likely to consent to demands'.

Passage X: question 39

Females are more likely to exhibit the characteristics of a 'tweenager' than males.

Answer: True

This is made quite clear in the passage: 'The branding and commercial appropriation (Russell and Tyler, 2002) of childhood, and especially female childhood' and later in the passage 'infantilisation of celebrity and especially young females'.

Passage X: question 40

Children aged 8 to 12 have only exhibited the characteristics of 'tweenagers' over the past ten years.

Answer: False

The passage states 'The terms "tweenies" and "tweenagers" have emerged within the last ten years to explain recent cultural changes in pre-teenage childhood cohort.' This does not mean that the characteristics of 'tweenagers' have emerged within the last ten years.

Passage XI: global studies

Passage XI: question 41

Students in full-time education in universities or colleges are not protected by the UNCRC.

Answer: False

The passage states 'The definition of a child under the convention is anyone under the age of 18'. It does not mention whether or not a child is in full-time education either at university or college. It is simply an age limitation and children under 18 may well be attending university or college.

Passage XI: question 42

The youth courts in Britain are more concerned with punishing children rather than rehabilitating them.

Answer: Can't Tell

The recent report to the UN inspectors claimed that Britain had a 'punitive juvenile justice system'. However, to make a more informed judgement about the statement, more information would be required as the report by the four Children's Commissioners is not elaborated on.

Passage XI: question 43

More children in Britain are physically abused by a parent or guardian than any other UNCRC signatory.

Answer: Can't Tell

The passage states the report to the UN inspectors stated 'public attitudes that demonise teenagers; lack of protection against physical punishment in the home and one of the highest levels of child poverty in Europe'. The passage does not provide comparative statistics of child abuse across the Convention's signatories.

Passage XI: question 44

There is a public perception in Britain today that adolescents are malevolent and evil.

Answer: True

The report to the UN inspectors relates to 'children and adolescents' and mentions the 'public attitudes that demonise teenagers'. Therefore there is a public perception that adolescents are malevolent and evil.

Chapter 9
The Quantitative Reasoning subtest

This chapter will help you to:

- understand the purpose and the format of quantitative reasoning tests;
- prepare for the Quantitative Reasoning subtest using general numerical aptitude questions;
- test your knowledge and understanding of numerical-type questions;
- identify those numerical skills where development is required.

Introduction

Pearson VUE describes the purpose of this subtest as follows.

> The Quantitative Reasoning subtest assesses a candidate's ability to solve numerical problems. This subtest requires the candidate to solve problems by extracting relevant information from tables and other numerical presentations. It assumes familiarity with numbers to a good pass at GCSE but the problems to be solved are less to do with numerical facility and more to do with problem solving (i.e. knowing what information to use and how to manipulate it using simple calculations and ratios). Hence it measures reasoning using numbers as a vehicle rather than measuring a facility with numbers.

As outlined in the introduction to this part of the book, commercially produced numerical aptitude tests have been in existence for many years, mainly for use in the selection and assessment of staff. There have been numerous books written on how to pass or how to master psychometric tests, and what follows is a précis on what you need to consider specifically in approaching the Quantitative Reasoning subtest. Essentially, the advice on preparation for any aptitude test, contained in the first chapter, holds true for numerical tests.

Quite simply, numerical tests are designed to measure your ability to understand numbers. This relates to the four basic arithmetic operations of addition, subtraction, multiplication and division, as well as number sequences and simple mathematics. Therefore, in preparing for such tests, you need to be able to perform simple calculations without the use of a calculator.

This chapter provides you with an opportunity to test your understanding and knowledge of the range of questions you are likely to be presented with in the UKCAT. By taking this opportunity you should be able to identify any numerical areas which you may need to develop. Obviously, as with any other type of examination, numerical questions can be presented in a variety of ways. However, the basic computations used will always be the same. So learn or remind yourself of the basics. The section following the subtest provides the answers to the questions. This includes not only the correct answer and rationale but also the reasons why the other options are incorrect. In addition, this section also provides the 'mathematical rule' for each question. All this is designed to reinforce or build on your understanding and knowledge of the syllabus areas.

Quantitative Reasoning subtest

For the purposes of this chapter, a range of questions have been designed to cover relevant areas of the Level 2 and Level 3 Adult Numeracy Core Curriculum produced by the Qualifications and Curriculum Authority. Level 3 is equivalent to GCSE standard, and a score of 27 or above (out of 36) on the practice test below equates to a Grade C or above at GCSE. This should be sufficient to deal with the scope of questions contained within the subtest. In reality, at this level, you should be getting all the questions correct.

The curriculum areas covered in the practice test are as follows.

- Basic arithmetic operations of addition, subtraction, multiplication and division.
- Powers and roots.
- Proportional change and ratios.
- Measurement of average and range to compare distributions, and estimate mean, median and range of grouped data.
- Conversion between fractions, decimals and percentages.
- Formulae, equations and expressions.
- Conversion of measurements between systems.

Response formats and example question

The type of format used in the Quantitative Reasoning subtest is the same as the one used as an example of multiple-choice questions in the introduction to this part of the book. That is, a *stem* in the form of a table, chart or graph, followed by a *lead-in question* and then five possible *choices* – A, B, C, D or E.

Example question

The following example requires you to select the correct answer from the five options provided. The rationale for the correct and incorrect answers is provided after the question.

The table below shows the miles travelled by a sales representative.

	Mon	Tue	Wed	Thu	Fri	Sat
WEEK 1	197.5	189	213.5	231	190	437
WEEK 2	116.5	145	202	173	52	

You want to find her median mileage over the 11 days. Which of these would you do?

A Find the sixth number and divide this by 2

B Add all the numbers together and divide by 11

C Rearrange the numbers into numerical order and then find the sixth number

D Find the average for each week and divide this by 2

E Add the two middle numbers together and divide this by 2

Median: rule

The median of a distribution is the middle value when the values are arranged in order. When there are two middle values (i.e. for an even number of values), you add the two middle numbers and divide by 2.

Answer C is correct: Rearrange the numbers into numerical order and then find the sixth number.

Rationale

There are 11 values, an odd number, so arrange the values into numerical order and then find the middle value, which is the sixth number, and this is the median.

A is incorrect: Find the sixth number and divide this by 2. Here there is an odd number of values so there is no need to divide anything by 2, only find the middle value.

B is incorrect: Add all the numbers together and divide by 11. This is the method for finding the mean, not the median.

D is incorrect: Find the average for each week and divide this by 2. This is not a method for finding any type of average.

E is incorrect: Add the two middle numbers together and divide this by 2. This is the method for finding the median when there is an even number of values.

Quantitative Reasoning practice subtest

The Quantitative Reasoning subtest consists of 36 items associated with tables, charts and/or graphs. A period of twenty-three minutes is allowed for the test, with one minute for instruction and twenty-two minutes for items.

If you want to simulate 'test conditions', you are advised to use rough paper to mark down your choice for each of the questions (i.e. A, B, C, D or E). The answers can then be checked against the 'answers' in the following section. Obviously, incorrect answers may identify a development need in a particular area of the curriculum. A simple on-screen calculator is available during the test.

Remember that each of the questions is always accompanied by five possible answers (A, B, C, D and E), and that only **one** answer is correct.

Also remember to read through all five competing answers before selecting what you consider to be the correct answer. By reading the four 'incorrect' answers you should confirm that your choice is in fact correct.

Questions 1 to 4 are about skyscrapers. Below are examples of the tallest skyscrapers across the USA with the height in metres shown in parenthesis:

Trump International Chicago (423)	Transamerica San Francisco (258)
Bank of America Atlanta (312)	Hancock Place Boston (241)
Devon Energy Oklahoma City (258)	Republic Plaza Denver (218)
Detroit Marriott Detroit (222)	JP Morgan Chase Houston (305)
Key Tower Cleveland (289)	Empire State Building New York (381)
IDS Tower Minneapolis (241)	Bank of America Houston (238)
RSA Battle House Mobile (227)	Columbia Centre Seattle (284)
Aon Centre Chicago (346)	John Hancock Centre Chicago (344)
30 Hudson Street Jersey City (238)	U.S. Steel Tower Pittsburgh (256)
Southeast Financial Centre Miami (233)	U.S. Bank Los Angeles (310)
Comcast Centre Philadelphia (297)	Chase Tower Indianapolis (253)
Bank of America Charlotte (265)	Bank of America Dallas (281)

1 What fraction of the skyscrapers are over 300 metres but less than 400 metres in height?

 A ½

 B ⅓

 C ¼

 D ⅕

 E ⅙

2 What is the ratio of skyscrapers that are greater than 258 metres high but less than 290 metres compared with skyscrapers that are less than 258 metres but greater than 220 metres?

 A 1:2

 B 2:3

 C 2:5

 D 3:7

 E 4:9

3 How many of the skyscrapers are less than 850 feet in height (1 metre = 3.3 feet)?

 A 4

 B 6

 C 8

 D 10

 E 12

4 What can you say that 25% of the skyscrapers are?

 A Less than 250 metres high

 B At least 230 metres but less than 250 metres high

 C More than 300 metres high

 D At least 290 metres but less than 350 metres high

 E At least 245 metres high

Questions 5 to 8 are about the following table that shows the average A-level raw score pass rates per subject area for students entering both redbrick universities and other universities

Redbrick universities	Pass rate	Other universities	Pass rate
English language	82	English language	78
English literature	75	English literature	63
Mathematics	88	Mathematics	76
History	69	History	72
Geography	72	Geography	65
Law	79	Law	58
Economics	66	Economics	71
French	87	French	67
German	82	German	71
Latin	64	Latin*	0

* Latin does not apply to other universities.

5 To the nearest round number, what is the mean average pass rate across all subjects for other universities?

A 9

B 69

C 78

D 138

E 621

6 What is the median average pass rate for redbrick universities?

A 71

B 75

C 77

D 79

E 88

7 What can you say about the range of the redbrick universities' average pass rates compared with the range of average pass rates of students entering the other universities?

   A The mode for the other universities is lower.

   B They are the same.

   C It is lower.

   D The median for the redbrick universities is higher.

   E It is higher.

8 What is the mode average pass rate of the redbrick universities?

   A 71

   B 72

   C 82

   D 85

   E 88

Questions 9 to 12 refer to the pie chart below, which groups the level of turnover of a number of organisations included in a business sector survey. The number of organisations per group is shown in parentheses.

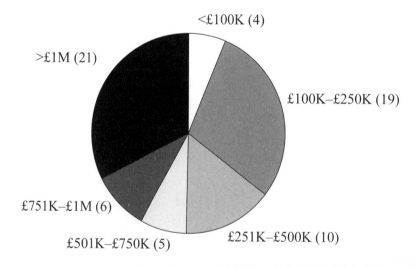

9 What percentage, to two decimal places, of organisations has a turnover in excess of £1M?

   A 49.53%

   B 46.34%

   C 32.31%

   D 57.89%

   E 62.16%

10 What is the ratio of the number of organisations with a turnover of £501K–£750K compared with the rest of the organisations?

   A 1:5

   B 4:9

   C 1:10

   D 1:12

   E 1:15

11 The Learning and Skills Council has asked the publishers of this business sector information also to produce the turnover of the organisations in euros. In converting pounds sterling to euros, where £1 = €1.45, what would be the lower limit of the range for those organisations with a turnover of £251K–£500K, in euros?

   A €145,000

   B €362,500

   C €363,950

   D €725,000

   E €726,450

12 The 65 organisations in this survey employ a total of 850 people of whom about 63% are employed by those organisations with a turnover in excess of £1M. The remaining employees are spread pro rata across the other organisations. How many employees, to the nearest round number, work for a company with a turnover of £251K–£500K?

A 7

B 12

C 15

D 19

E 26

Questions 13 to 16 relate to the table below that shows the average gross weekly earnings by UK country.

Year	United Kingdom	England	Wales	Scotland	Northern Ireland
1999	407.8	414.9	358.7	377.0	352.4
2000	425.1	433.3	372.8	388.6	367.6
2001	449.7	459.2	385.8	411.1	381.5
2002	472.1	482.0	405.2	434.6	396.8
2003	487.1	497.2	421.8	447.0	411.5
2004	498.2	508.1	438.3	455.5	430.9
2005	516.4	525.5	454.8	479.0	450.7
2006	534.9	544.3	466.2	499.7	469.4
2007	550.3	560.8	472.0	514.6	471.7
2008	575.6	586.7	498.2	536.3	487.0
2009	587.2	597.4	506.3	555.1	509.1
2010	598.3	608.6	516.0	570.1	511.6

13 Which country, including the United Kingdom, had the highest range of average gross weekly earnings between 1999 and 2010?

A Wales

B Northern Ireland

C United Kingdom

D Scotland

E England

14 Which one of the following statements is supported by the information contained in the table?

A   In 2002 Wales's average gross weekly earnings were approximately 10% less than those in England.

B   Scotland has the third highest average gross weekly earnings in the country.

C   In 2010 Northern Ireland's average gross annual earnings will be over $\frac{1}{10}$ less than the average UK earnings.

D   Compared to 1999, in 2010 the difference in average gross weekly earnings between England and Scotland has decreased.

E   Northern Ireland's average gross weekly earnings exceeded those of Wales in three separate years.

15 What is the percentage increase (to one decimal place) of the average gross weekly earnings in the United Kingdom between 1999 and 2010?

A   28.9%

B   31.8%

C   40.7%

D   46.7%

E   51.2%

16 What is the approximate ratio of the average gross weekly earnings of Northern Ireland in 2004 compared to the country's earnings in 2010?

A   1:2

B   1:3

C   2:3

D   3:4

E   4:5

Questions 17 to 20 are about the table on page 102, which is being used by a group of 12 people forming a diet club. They have agreed to use a calorie count method and have produced the table showing the serving size, calorie count and grams of fat for bread, biscuits, cakes, eggs and dairy products.

Item	Serving size (grams)	Calorie count	Grams of fat
Bagel	85	216	1.4
Baguette	150	360	1.8
Chocolate cake	34	180	10.4
Biscuit	15	74	3.3
Danish pastry	67	287	17.4
Doughnut	49	140	2.0
Hot cross bun	70	205	3.9
Jaffa cake	12	46	1.0
Scone	70	225	17.6
White crusty roll	50	140	1.2
Brown bread	25	74	0.7
Granary bread	25	59	0.7
Pitta bread	25	147	1.1
White bread	37	84	0.6
Wholemeal bread	36	79	1.0
Toast	33	88	0.6
Butter	10	74	8.2
Cheddar cheese	40	172	14.8
Cream cheese	34	58	4.8
Eggs size 3	57	84	6.2

17 The estimated average requirements are a daily calorie intake of 1940 calories per day for women and 2550 for men. The group agrees to follow the same daily menu that provides for an intake of 1940 calories. The men then select items to take them up to their recommended calorie intake. One of the men decides he will achieve this by just eating one serving size bagel and butter and as much toast as he is allowed where a serving of 33 grams equates to one slice of toast.

What is the maximum number of slices of toast the man may have to stay under the recommended calorie limit?

A   3 slices

B   4 slices

C   7 slices

D   9 slices

E   11 slices

The group categorises the items of food into low to high calorie content and produces the following table.

Calorie count per serving	Number of items
<80	7
>80 but <109	3
>109 but <149	3
>149 but <189	2
189 and over	6

The group then checks its table.

18 Is there anything wrong with the total number of items in the table?

A   One too few of calorie count >149 but <189

B   Two too many of calorie count <80

C   One too many of calorie count 189 and over

D   Total number of calorie count correct

E   One too few of calorie count >109 but <149

19 A group member wants to ascertain the median calorie count for all the items in the table. Which one of the following should he do?

A   Re-arrange the numbers into numerical order, find the tenth number and divide by 2.

B   Add all the numbers together and divide by 20.

C   Find the average of all the numbers and divide by 2.

D   Find the calorie count number that occurs most frequently.

E   Re-arrange the numbers into numerical order, add the tenth and eleventh numbers and divide by 2.

20 It is the birthday of one of the group and another member wants to buy a chocolate cake, large enough for each member to have one serving size. However, before going shopping she wants to know what weight of cake she will need for the group, measured in ounces. Grams are converted to ounces by dividing grams by 28.3.

If X is the weight of the required cake in ounces, and G is the weight of one serving size in grams, which one of the following options is the correct formula?

A $X = 12 \left(\frac{G}{28.3}\right)$

B $G = \frac{12X}{28.3}$

C $G = \frac{12}{28.3X}$

D $X = 28.3 \left(\frac{G}{12}\right)$

E $X = \frac{28.3}{12G}$

Questions 21 to 24 relate to the following information about the Links View Golf and Country Club, which provides tailor-made stays for those wishing to use the facilities of either their two 18-hole championship golf courses or the spa complex and treatment centre.

The table below shows the golf packages currently being offered.

Packages	Cost	Breakfast	Dinner	Offer includes
Stay & Play 1 night (Mon–Thurs)	£129*	YES	YES	2 rounds of golf on either course
Stay & Play 1 night (Fri–Sat)	£139*	YES	YES	2 rounds of golf on either course
Stay & Play Sunday Special 1 night only	£129*	YES	YES	All day golf pass for 2 days
Stay & Play 2 nights (Mon–Thurs)	£209*	YES	YES	3 rounds of golf on either course

Stay & Play 2 nights (Fri–Sat)	£229*	YES	YES	3 rounds of golf on either course
Stay & Play 3 nights (Mon–Thurs)	£259*	YES	YES	4 rounds of golf on either course
Stay & Play 3 nights (Fri–Sun)	£289*	YES	YES	4 rounds of golf on either course

* Price per person based on two sharing – add £20 supplement for single room occupancy
* Deduct £5 per person per night for Fairways & Bunkers lodge rooms

21 A golf society comprising three couples and two single people (not sharing) has decided to stay at the Golf and Country Club, arriving at lunchtime on a Friday. One of the couples and one of the singles plan to stay one night only and the remainder will stay for two nights. Those staying one night wish to be accommodated in the lodge rooms.

What would be the total cost for the golf society?

A £1,607.00

B £1,587.00

C £1,602.00

D £1,507.00

E £1,547.00

22 Discounting the supplements, what is the range of prices of the packages offered by the Golf and Country Club?

A £129.00

B £139.00

C £160.00

D £198.00

E £209.00

23 From January to April the Golf and Country Club has a special winter deal offering a discount on its golf packages if combined with a spa and treatments package. For a three-night stay (Fri–Sun) the spa package, which is normally £75 per couple, has been discounted by 5%, and there is a 15% discount on the golf package.

Two couples decide to take advantage of this offer. How much would the special winter deal cost them, per person, to the nearest whole number?

A £281.00

B £283.00

C £246.00

D £317.00

E £327.00

24 The spa complex offers the following treatments: facials and skin treatments; health massage; *cellulite and body contouring; pedicure and manicure; facial thread vein treatment; *reiki; crystal therapy; reflexology; and aromatherapy. All treatments cost £37.95, and – apart from those marked with an asterisk – all are currently available on a 3 for 2 basis.

Two women decide to use the spa complex facilities. One woman decides to have the pedicure, crystal therapy and reflexology, and the other woman decides to have the health massage, reiki and crystal therapy. It is one woman's birthday and the other woman decides to pay for her treatments as a gift, as well as paying for her own.

If she set aside £250.00, how much money would she have left after paying for all the treatments?

A £174.10

B £136.15

C £98.20

D £60.25

E £22.30

Questions 25 to 28 relate to the chart on the opposite page, which shows the results of the final of the pole vault competition at an athletics meeting. The heights shown are in metres; S = successful vault and F = failed vault. Competitors who have three failed attempts at a height are eliminated.

	4.2	4.4	4.6	4.8	5.0	5.2	5.4	5.6	5.8	6.0
Tully	S	S	S	S	S	S	S	FS	FS	FFF
Roberts	S	FS	FFS	FFF	–	–	–	–	–	–
Abada	S	S	FS	FFS	FFF	–	–	–	–	–
Walker	S	FS	S	FS	FFS	FS	FFS	FFF	–	–
Burgess	S	S	FS	S	FS	FS	FFF	–	–	–
Bubka	S	S	S	S	S	S	S	S	S	FS
Hartwig	FS	FS	FS	FS	FS	FFS	FS	FFS	FFF	–
Mack	S	FS	FFF	–	–	–		–		
Mesnil	S	S	S	FS	FS	FFS	FFS	FFF	–	–
Markov	S	S	FS	FS	FFS	S	FS	FFS	FFF	–
Smith	S	S	FS	S	FS	FFS	FFF	–	–	–
Seagren	S	S	S	FS	S	FS	FFS	FS	FFS	FFF

25 What percentage of competitors, to the nearest whole number, had a failed vault when the bar was set at 4.6 metres?

A 33%

B 42%

C 50%

D 58%

E 67%

26 Before the bar was raised to 4.8 metres what number of failed vaults had occurred compared to the total number of vaults, expressed as a fraction?

A ¼

B ⅓

C ½

D ²⁄₉

E ³⁄₁₀

27 When the bar was set at 5.2 metres, what ratio of competitors had more than one failed vault compared to those remaining in the competition?

A   1:2

B   1:3

C   1:4

D   2:3

E   3:4

28 For all the competitors in this final, what is the average greatest height successfully vaulted, to one decimal place?

A   5.0 metres

B   5.1 metres

C   5.2 metres

D   5.3 metres

E   5.4 metres

Questions 29 to 32 are based on the table below that details the deals available from broadband providers.

Provider	Speed	Downloads	Contract	Cost (monthly)
Chat-Chat	20MB	20GB	12 months	£12.00
Yellow	24MB	unlimited	12 months	£12.50
E20	24MB	40GB	18 months	£7.50
Pure Media	24MB	unlimited	12 months	£12.00
DTT	20MB	40GB	18 months	£15.00

All the providers except **E20** have 'special' offers for new customers: **Chat-Chat** – 40% reduction for 6 months; **Yellow** – first 3 months free; **Pure Media** – £40.00 off; **DTT** – £1.00 a month for first 3 months.

29 Irrespective of the speed, downloads and contract period which one of the providers would be the cheapest over the first 6 months?

   A Chat-Chat

   B Yellow

   C E20

   D Pure Media

   E DTT

30 Ignoring special offers which one of the following statements is true?

   A Only providers with unlimited downloads have 24MB speed.

   B The mean average monthly contract cost of the five providers to the nearest £ is £12.00.

   C There is a 50% cost difference in the providers who only offer an 18 months contract.

   D The monthly contract cost of providers with 20GB downloads is less than those having 40GB downloads.

   E Providers who offer 20MB speeds require an 18 months contract.

31 When considering an 18 months contract with either E20 or DTT, expressed as a percentage (to the nearest whole number), how much more would it cost to use DTT instead of E20?

   A 47%

   B 60%

   C 69%

   D 77%

   E 85%

32 Where a person wants a minimum 24MB speed, 40GB for downloads and a 12 months contract, taking into account the special offers for new customers, what would be the actual price of the cheapest provider over the 12 months?

A £104.00

B £112.50

C £138.00

D £144.00

E £150.00

Questions 33 to 36 relate to merchant ships and boats. When travelling on the water, distance is measured in nautical miles (nm) and speed in knots (kts).

33 A merchant vessel leaves Liverpool port (UK) at 0900 hours on Monday 1 March en route to Bilbao port (Spain). The distance between the two ports is 1,138 miles. The average cruising speed of the merchant vessel on this journey is 15 knots.

What time, day and date does the vessel arrive at Bilbao port to the nearest hour? (1 knot = 1.15 miles per hour; Bilbao port is UK time + 1 hour.)

A   1800 hours, Wednesday 3 March

B   0200 hours, Thursday 4 March

C   0300 hours, Thursday 4 March

D   0400 hours, Thursday 4 March

E   1400 hours, Thursday 4 March

34 Johnson has entered her 'firebrand' dinghy in a race being held in her twin town of La Rochelle in France organised by the local yacht club. The race consists of completing a course measuring 3 kilometres marked out by a series of orange buoys. She decides to practise the course the day before the race. The wind is difficult with gusts and calms in almost equal measure. In sailing the course Johnson manages an average speed of 3 knots for 10 minutes, 10 knots for 20 minutes and 7 knots for 30 minutes.

How many laps of the marked course did Johnson complete, to one decimal place? (1 knot = 1.852 kilometres per hour (km/h))

A   3.5 laps

B   4.5 laps

C   6.0 laps

D   6.7 laps

E   12.3 laps

35 A cruise ship is powered by an oil turbine with an average oil usage of 10 litres of oil per 4 nautical miles (nm) travelled. The capacity of oil that can be stored on the ship is 7,500 litres. The ship is currently 42% of the way through its cruise round the Caribbean islands. The distance back to the ship's home quay is 768 nm. What percentage of oil will be in the ship's storage tank when it arrives at its home quay if the oil tank was 68% full at the time of departure?

A   7%

B   14%

C   15%

D   18%

E   24%

36 A French ferry travels between Dunkerque and Dover, making four return trips each weekday, and five on each day of the weekend. The distance between Dunkerque and Dover is 70 miles. The ferry has a fuel capacity of 1,200 litres and on average travels 5 miles for each litre of fuel. Fuel costs in the UK are 54p per litre. In France the cost of one litre of fuel is 2.5% cheaper than in the UK due to less VAT being paid.

What is the value, in euros, of the fuel remaining in the tank at the end of one week where the tank was full at the outset? (£1 = €1.16)

A   €164.97

B   €169.20

C   €221.13

D   €226.80

E   €232.47

Quantitative Reasoning practice subtest: answers

Question number	Correct response	Question number	Correct response
1	C	19	E
2	B	20	A
3	D	21	B
4	D	22	C
5	B	23	A
6	C	24	D
7	E	25	D
8	C	26	E
9	C	27	B
10	D	28	D
11	C	29	D
12	A	30	B
13	E	31	C
14	C	32	A
15	D	33	D
16	E	34	B
17	A	35	E
18	C	36	C

Quantitative Reasoning practice subtest: explanation of answers

Question 1

Fractions: rule

To find one number as a **fraction** of the other, you write the numbers as a fraction, with the first number on the top and the second number on the bottom. The top line of a fraction is called the numerator and the bottom line of a fraction is called the denominator.

Answer C is correct: $\frac{1}{4}$.

Rationale

Step 1: there is a total of 24 skyscrapers, so this number goes on the bottom as the denominator.

Step 2: there are 6 skyscrapers between 300 and 400 metres, so this number goes on the top as the numerator.

Step 3: the fraction is therefore $\frac{6}{24}$.

Step 4: this fraction can be cancelled down as both the numerator and denominator are divisible by 6, so the fraction is $\frac{1}{4}$.

Answer A is incorrect: $\frac{1}{2}$. For this answer to be correct the number of skyscrapers between 300 and 400 metres would need to be 12, so $\frac{12}{24}$ which can be cancelled down to $\frac{1}{2}$.

Answer B is incorrect: $\frac{1}{3}$. For this answer to be correct the number of skyscrapers between 300 and 400 metres would need to be 8, so $\frac{8}{24}$ which can be cancelled down to $\frac{1}{3}$.

Answer D is incorrect: $\frac{1}{5}$. This answer could not be obtained from the parameters of the question. The only fraction possible where the number of skyscrapers between 300 and 400 metres was 5 would be $\frac{5}{24}$.

Answer E is incorrect: $\frac{1}{6}$. For this answer to be correct the number of skyscrapers between 300 and 400 metres would need to be 4, so $\frac{4}{24}$ which can be cancelled down to $\frac{1}{6}$.

Question 2

Less than, less than or equal to, greater than, greater than or equal to: rule; Conversion: rule

Less than n does not include n.
Less than or equal to n does include n.
Greater than n does not include n.
Greater than or equal to n does include n

Ratio: rule

A **ratio** allows one quantity to be compared with another quantity. Any two numbers can be compared by writing them alongside each other with the numbers separated by a ratio sign (:).

Answer B is correct: 2:3.

Rationale

Step 1: there are 6 skyscrapers 258 metres high but less than 290 metres.

Step 2: there are 9 skyscrapers less than 258 metres but higher than 220 metres.

Step 3: write the figures separated by a ratio sign (:) with the lower number being compared first, so here 6:9.

Step 4: cancel these figures down if possible, so both can be divided by 3 to give 2:3.

Answer A is incorrect: 1:2. We know the number of skyscrapers that are 258 metres high but less than 290 metres is 6 and 1 can be a factor of that number. However, the number of skyscrapers less than 258 metres but higher than 220 metres is 9 and since 2 cannot be a factor of 9 the ratio cannot be 1:2.

Answer C is incorrect: 2:5. We know the number of skyscrapers that are 258 metres high but less than 290 metres is 6 and 2 can be a factor of that number. However, the number of skyscrapers less than 258 metres but higher than 220 metres is 9 and since 5 cannot be a factor of 9 the ratio cannot be 2:5.

Answer D is incorrect: 3:7. We know the number of skyscrapers that are 258 metres high but less than 290 metres is 6 and 3 can be a factor of that number. However, the number of skyscrapers less than 258 metres but higher than 220 metres is 9 and since 7 cannot be a factor of 9 the ratio cannot be 3:7.

Answer E is incorrect: 4:9. We know the number of skyscrapers that are 258 metres high but less than 290 metres is 6 and 4 cannot be a factor of that number therefore that ratio cannot be 4:9.

Question 3

Conversion: rule

The **conversion** is the equation for converting metres to feet (1 metre – 3.3 feet).

Answer D is correct: 10.

Rationale

Step 1: convert 850 feet to metres, $\frac{850}{3.3} = 257.58$ metres

Step 2: from the table identify the number of skyscrapers below 257.58 metres = 10

Answer A is incorrect: 4. For this answer to be correct the number of skyscrapers would have needed to be less than 770 feet in height.

Answer B is incorrect: 6. For this answer to be correct the number of skyscrapers would have needed to be less than 786 feet in height.

Answer C is incorrect: 8. For this answer to be correct the number of skyscrapers would have needed to be less than 796 feet in height.

Answer E is incorrect: 12. For this answer to be correct the number of skyscrapers would have needed to be less than 852 feet in height.

Question 4

Percentages: rule
To express one number as a percentage of another, write the first number as a fraction of the second and convert the fraction to a percentage by multiplying by 100.

Answer D is correct: At least 290 metres but less than 350 metres high.

Rationale
Step 1: in this instance we are given a percentage, i.e. 25% of the total number of skyscrapers, so we can find the number of skyscrapers as a percentage of the whole.

Step 2: 25% of $24 = \frac{24}{100} \times 25 = 6$, there are 6 skyscrapers between 290 and 350 metres.

Answer A is incorrect: Less than 250 metres high. There are 8 skyscrapers that are less than 250 metres high.

Answer B is incorrect: At least 230 metres but less than 250 metres high. There are 5 skyscrapers at least 230 metres but less than 250 metres.

Answer C is incorrect: More than 300 metres high. There are 7 skyscrapers that are more than 300 metres high.

Answer E is incorrect: At least 245 metres high. There are 8 skyscrapers that are at least 245 metres high.

Question 5

Mean: rule
The **mean** (or arithmetic mean) of a distribution is found by summing the values of the distribution and dividing by the number of values.

Answer B is correct: 69.

Rationale
Step 1: mean = sum of values ÷ number of values.

Step 2: $\dfrac{58 + 63 + 65 + 67 + 71 + 71 + 72 + 76 + 78}{9}$

Step 3: mean = $\frac{621}{9}$ = 69.

Answer A is incorrect: 9. This is the number of values in the distribution of the other universities and not the mean.

Answer C is incorrect: 78. This is the extreme upper value of the other universities, i.e. the highest subject average pass rate of the other universities, and not the mean.

Answer D is incorrect: 138. This is the sum of the value (621) divided by half the number of values (4.5) whereas the number of values is actually 9.

Answer E is incorrect: 621. This is the sum of the values; it needs to be divided by the number of values, which is 9, to find the mean.

Question 6

Median: rule
The **median** of a distribution is the middle value when the values are arranged in order. When there are two middle values (i.e. for an even number of values), then you add the two numbers and divide by 2.

Answer C is correct: 77.

Rationale
Step 1: arrange the values in order so 64, 66, 69, 72, 75, 79, 82, 82, 87, 88.

Step 2: there is an even number of values so the median is $\frac{75 + 79}{2}$ = 77, as 75 and 79 are the 'middle' values in the distribution.

Answer A is incorrect: 71. This is the middle value, the median average pass rate, of the other universities.

Answer B is incorrect: 75. This is the fifth value in the distribution and not the middle value; the median is halfway between 75 and 79.

Answer D is incorrect: 79. This is the sixth value in the distribution and not the middle value; the median is halfway between 75 and 79.

Answer E is incorrect: 88. This is simply the highest average pass rate.

Question 7

Range: rule

The **range** of a distribution is found by working out the difference between the highest value and the lowest value. The range should always be given as a single value.

Answer E is correct: It is higher.

Rationale

Step 1: redbrick universities' greatest value = 88. Lowest value = 64. The range = greatest value – lowest value = 88 – 64 = 24.

Step 2: other universities' greatest value = 78. Lowest value = 58. The range = greatest value – lowest value = 78 – 58 = 20.

Step 3: therefore the range of the redbrick universities' average pass rates is higher than that of the other universities.

Answer A is incorrect: The mode for the other universities is lower. This answer is incorrect as the mode is irrelevant to calculating the range.

Answer B is incorrect: They are the same. The range of the redbrick universities is 24 and the range of other universities is 20, therefore the ranges are not the same.

Answer C is incorrect: It is lower. The range of redbrick universities is greater than the range of other universities, therefore this option is incorrect.

Answer D is incorrect: The median for the redbrick universities is higher. This answer is incorrect as the median is irrelevant to calculating the range.

Question 8

Mode: rule

The **mode** is the number in a distribution that has the highest frequency; that is, it appears the most times in a collection of values.

Answer C is correct: 82.

Rationale

The value 82 appears the most times (twice) in the list of redbrick universities' average pass rates.

Answer A is incorrect: 71. This value is the mode for the other universities, appearing twice in the list of average pass rates.

Answer B is incorrect: 72. This value appears in the list of redbrick universities' average pass rates but it only appears once. 72 also appears once in the list of other universities but cannot be calculated within the rule as the two lists are separate.

Answer D is incorrect: 85. This value does not appear at all in the list of average pass rates for redbrick universities.

Answer E is incorrect: 88. This is simply the highest value in the list of average pass rates for redbrick universities but is not the mode.

Question 9

Percentages: rule

To express one number as a **percentage** of another, write the first number as a fraction of the second and convert the fraction to a percentage by multiplying it by 100.

Answer C is correct: 32.31%.

Rationale

Step 1: the number of organisations with a turnover in excess of £1M = 21. The number of organisations in the sample = 65.

Step 2: 21 as a fraction of 65 = $\frac{21}{65}$

Step 3: convert to a percentage, so $\frac{21}{65} \times 100 = 32.31\%$.

Step 4: therefore 32.31% of the organisations have a turnover in excess of £1M.

Answer A is incorrect: 49.53%. Using approximations, we know that 50 per cent of something is half of it and half of 65 is approximately 33, so this cannot be the correct answer as we know the number of organisations with a turnover in excess of £1M is 21 and therefore a percentage figure considerably less than 50 per cent.

Answer B is incorrect: 46.34%. Using approximations, we know that 50 per cent of something is half of it and half of 65 is approximately 33, so this cannot be the correct answer as the number of organisations with a turnover in excess of £1M is 21 and therefore a percentage figure less than 50 per cent. However, this option would have to be calculated to ensure the answer was incorrect.

Answer D is incorrect: 57.89%. Using approximations, we know that 50 per cent of something is half of it and half of 65 is approximately 33. There are 21 organisations with a turnover in excess of £1M, so the answer must be under 50 per cent.

Answer E is incorrect: 62.16%. Using approximations, we know that 50 per cent of something is half of it and half of 65 is approximately 33, so this cannot be the correct answer as the number of organisations with a turnover in excess of £1M is 21 and therefore a percentage considerably under 50 per cent.

Question 10

Ratios: rule

A **ratio** allows one quantity to be compared with another quantity. Any two numbers can be compared by writing them alongside each other with the numbers separated by a ratio sign (:).

Answer D is correct: 1:12.

Rationale

Step 1: five organisations have a turnover of £501K–£750K and therefore 65 – 5 = 60 organisations have a different turnover.

Step 2: write the figures separated by the ratio sign with the number being compared first, so here 5:60.

Step 3: cancel these figures down if possible. Both can be divided by 5 to give 1:12.

Step 4: the ratio of the number of organisations with a turnover of £501K–£750K compared with the rest of the organisations is 1:12.

Answer A is incorrect: 1:5. Multiplying both sides of this ratio by 5 gives 5:25 and so this option cannot be correct, as the ratio is 5:60.

Answer B is incorrect: 4:9. Multiplying both sides of this ratio by 5 gives 20:45 and so this option cannot be correct, as the ratio is 5:60.

Answer C is incorrect: 1:10. Multiplying both sides of this ratio by 5 gives 5:50 and so this option cannot be correct, as the ratio is 5:60.

Answer E is incorrect: 1:15. Multiplying both sides of this ratio by 5 gives 5:75 and so this option cannot be correct, as the ratio is 5:60.

Question 11

Conversion: rule

The equation for **converting** pounds to euros is $€ = £ \times 1.45$.

Answer C is correct: €363,950.

Rationale

Step 1: $€ = £ \times 1.45$.

Step 2: substitute £ with 251,000, so $€ = 251,000 \times 1.45$.

Step 3: $€ = 363,950$.

Answer A is incorrect: €145,000. This conversion is from £100K (i.e. € = 100,000 × 1.45 = €145,000).

Answer B is incorrect: €362,500. This conversion is from £250K (i.e. € = 250,000 × 1.45 = €362,500).

Answer D is incorrect: €725,000. This conversion is from £500K (i.e. € = 500,000 × 1.45 = €725,000).

Answer E is incorrect: €726,450. This conversion is from £501K (i.e. € = 501,000 × 1.45 = €726,450).

Question 12

Percentage and proportion: rule

To find the **percentage** of an amount, find 1% of the amount and then multiply to get the required amount. This question also contains **subtraction** and **division**.

Answer A is correct: 7.

Rationale

Step 1: find 1% of the amount $\left(\frac{850}{100} = 8.5\right)$.

Step 2: multiply by the percentage required (8.5 × 63 = 535.5).

Step 3: find the remaining number of employees (850 − 535.5 = 314.5).

Step 4: divide the remaining employees by the number of other organisations $\left(\frac{314.5}{44} = 7.14\right)$ which, to the nearest round number, is 7.

Answer B is incorrect: 12. This answer is incorrect as the number of employees working for organisations with a turnover in excess of £1M (535.5) has been divided by the number of other organisations (44), instead of dividing the remaining number of employees (314.5) by 44.

Answer C is incorrect: 15. This answer is incorrect as the number of remaining employees (314.5) has been divided by the number of organisations with a turnover in excess of £1M (21).

Answer D is incorrect: 19. This answer is incorrect as it has taken the total number of employees (850) and divided by the number of other organisations (44).

Answer E is incorrect: 26. This answer is incorrect as the number of employees working for organisations with a turnover in excess of £1M (535.5) has been divided by the number of those organisations (21).

Question 13

Range: rule

The range of a distribution is found by working out the difference between the highest value and the lowest value. The range should always be given as a single value.

Answer E is correct: England.

Rationale

Step 1: in relation to England the highest value in the distribution is 608.6 and the lowest value is 414.9.

Step 2: the difference between the highest and lowest value is 608.6 – 414.9 = 193.7.

Answer A is incorrect: Wales. The highest value is 516.0 and the lowest value is 358.7, so 516.0 – 358.7 = 157.3. The range for Wales could have been discounted early on due to the obvious difference in the highest and lowest values compared to the three 'highest' answers.

Answer B is incorrect: Northern Ireland. The highest value is 511.6 and the lowest value is 352.4, so 511.6 – 352.4 = 159.2. Similar to Wales, Northern Ireland could have been discounted early on due to the obvious difference in the highest and lowest values compared to the three 'highest' answers.

Answer C is incorrect: United Kingdom. The highest value is 598.3 and the lowest value is 407.8, so 598.3 – 407.8 = 190.5.

Answer D is incorrect: Scotland. The highest value is 570.1 and the lowest value is 377.0, so 570.1 – 377.0 = 193.1.

Question 14

Interpreting data: rule

When interpreting data, this may involve identifying information presented in some form of pictorial or visual display.

Answer C is correct: In 2010 Northern Ireland's average gross annual earnings will be over $\frac{1}{10}$ less than the average UK earnings.

Rationale

Step 1: in 2010 the average gross weekly earnings were 598.3 (UK) and 511.6 (Northern Ireland).

Step 2: find the percentage difference, 598.3 − 511.6 − 86.7, so $\frac{86.7}{598.3}$ x 100 = 14.49% (14.5%).

Step 3: 14.5% as a fraction is $\frac{14.5}{100}$; $\frac{1}{10}$ is $\frac{10}{100}$, so the earnings will be over $\frac{1}{10}$ less than the average UK earnings. The word 'annual' is a distracter in the statement.

Answer A is incorrect: In 2002 Wales's average gross weekly earnings were approximately 10% less than those in England. In 2002 average gross weekly earnings in England were 482.0 and in Wales were 405.8. 10% of 482.0 = $\frac{482.0}{100}$ x 10 = 48.2; 482.0 − 48.2 = 433.8.

Answer B is incorrect: Scotland has the third highest average gross weekly earnings in the country. The table shows that England with 608.6 is the highest and that Scotland with 570.1 is the second highest. Obviously the UK figures can be discounted.

Answer D is incorrect: Compared to 1999, in 2010 the difference in average gross weekly earnings between England and Scotland has decreased. The earnings gap in 1999 was 414.9 (England) − 377.0 (Scotland) = 37.9 and in 2010 was 608.6 (England) − 570.1 (Scotland) = 38.5, so the gap has increased by 0.6.

Answer E is incorrect: Northern Ireland's average gross weekly earnings exceeded those of Wales in three separate years. The table indicates that Northern Ireland's average gross weekly earnings only exceeded Wales in two separate years, i.e. 2006 and 2009.

Question 15

Percentage change: rule
To work out the **percentage change**, work out the increase or decrease and divide it by the original amount, then multiply by 100. Percentage change = (change ÷ original amount) x 100, where the change may be an increase, decrease, profit, loss, error, etc.

Answer D is correct: 46.7%.

Rationale
Step 1: gather the information. In 1999 the average gross weekly earnings in the UK were 407.8 and in 2010 were 598.3.

Step 2: the increase between 1999 and 2010 is 598.3 − 407.8 = 190.5.

Step 3: the percentage increase is $\frac{190.5}{407.8}$ × 100 = 46.71, to one decimal place 46.7.

Answer A is incorrect: 28.9%. This answer has taken the increase of the 2000 and 2010 averages instead of the 1999 and 2010 averages and also divided the increase by the 2010 figure. This gives a calculation of 598.3 − 425.1 = 173.2, and shows the percentage increase as $\frac{173.2}{598.3}$ × 100 = 28.9%.

Answer B is incorrect: 31.8%. This answer has divided the increase by the 2010 figure instead of the 1999 figure. This gives a calculation of 598.3 – 407.8 = 190.5 and shows the percentage increase as $\frac{190.5}{598.3} \times 100 = 31.8\%$.

Answer C is incorrect: 40.7%. This answer has taken the increase of the 2000 and 2010 averages instead of the 1999 and 2010 averages. This gives a calculation of 598.3 – 425.1 = 173.2, so that the percentage increase is $\frac{173.2}{425.1} \times 100 = 40.7\%$.

Answer E is incorrect: 71.2%. This answer has incorrectly transposed the UK 2010 figure as 698.3 instead of 598.3. This gives a calculation of 698.3 – 407.8 = 290.5, so that the percentage increase is $\frac{290.5}{407.8} \times 100 = 71.2\%$.

Question 16

Ratio: rule
A **ratio** allows one quantity to be compared with another quantity. Any two numbers can be compared by writing them alongside each other with the numbers separated by a ratio sign (:).

Answer E is correct: 4:5.

Rationale
Step 1: in 2004 the average gross weekly earnings in Northern Ireland were 430.9 and in 2010 were 511.6.

Step 2: write the figures separated by a ratio sign (:) with the lower number being compared first, so here 430.9:511.6.

Step 3: use approximation so the ratio is 430.9:511.6 or 43:51 or 40:50.

Step 4: cancel these figures down if possible; both are divisible by 10 to give an approximate ratio of 4:5.

Answer A is incorrect: 1:2. The figures provided in the table for Northern Ireland would not allow a ratio of 1:2.

Answer B is incorrect: 1:3. The figures provided in the table for Northern Ireland would not allow a ratio of 1:3.

Answer C is incorrect: 2:3. The figures provided in the table for Northern Ireland would not allow a ratio of 2:3.

Answer D is incorrect: 3:4. The figures provided in the table for Northern Ireland would not allow a ratio of 3:4.

Question 17

Interpreting data: rule

When **interpreting data**, this may involve identifying information presented in some form of pictorial or visual display.

Answer A is correct: 3 slices.

Rationale

Step 1: calculate the maximum number of calories the man can use, i.e. 2550 – 1940 = 610.

Step 2: calculate the calorie intake of one serving size bagel and butter, i.e. 216 + 74 = 290.

Step 3: calculate the number of calories the man can use after the bagel and butter is subtracted from his allowance, i.e. 610 – 290 = 320.

Step 4: therefore the maximum number of slices the man will be allowed is 320 divided by 88 (calorie count for toast), i.e. $\frac{320}{88}$ = 3.6 slices.

Answer B is incorrect: 4 slices. This answer has only subtracted the calorie count for the bagel in Step 2 above and then divided by 88, i.e. $\frac{394}{88}$ = 4.5 slices.

Answer C is incorrect: 7 slices. This is a purely random answer and has no basis in any calculations.

Answer D is incorrect: 9 slices. This has correctly calculated the calorie count in Step 3 above but has then divided this by 33, the serving size in grams, and not the calorie count, i.e. $\frac{320}{33}$ = 9.7 slices.

Answer E is incorrect: 11 slices. As with answer B, this has subtracted the calorie count for the bagel only but in addition has divided the remainder by 33 (serving size in grams) and not the calorie count, i.e. $\frac{394}{33}$ = 11.9 slices.

Question 18

Interpreting data: rule

When **interpreting data**, this may involve identifying information presented in some form of pictorial or visual display.

Answer C is correct: One too many of calorie count 189 and over.

Rationale

Step 1: sum the number of items in the first table, which is 20.

Step 2: sum the number of items in the second table, which is 7 + 3 + 3 + 2 + 6 = 21.

Step 3: 21 – 20 = +1, therefore there is one too many in the second table. Checking against each category reveals that calorie count 189 and over has 6 instead of 5 items.

Answer A is incorrect: One too few of calorie count >149 but < 189. There is one too many items in the second table and not one too few.

Answer B is incorrect: Two too many of calorie count <80. There is only one too many items in the second table, not two too many.

Answer D is incorrect: Total number of calorie count correct. There is one too many items in the second table, therefore this statement is incorrect.

Answer E is incorrect: One too few of calorie count >109 but <149. There is one too many items missing from the second table and not one too few.

Question 19

Median: Rule
The **median** of a distribution is the middle value when the values are arranged in order. When there are two middle values (i.e. for an even number of values) then you add the two middle numbers and divide by 2.

Answer E is correct: Re-arrange the numbers into numerical order, add the tenth and eleventh numbers and divide by 2.

Rationale
The median of a distribution is the middle value when the values are arranged in order. In the table there are 20 separate values and therefore the sum of the tenth and eleventh numbers, divided by 2, is the median.

Answer A is incorrect: Re-arrange the numbers into numerical order, find the tenth number and divide by 2. Here there is an even number of values so you need to find the two middle numbers (tenth and eleventh), add them together and divide them by 2.

Answer B is incorrect: Add all the numbers together and divide by 20. This is the method for finding the mean, not the median.

Answer C is incorrect: Find the average of all the numbers and divide by 2. This is not a method for finding any type of average.

Answer D is incorrect: Find the calorie count number that occurs most frequently. This is the method for finding the mode, not the median.

Question 20

Substitution: rule
Substitution means that you replace the letters in a formula or expression by the given number.

Answer A is correct: $X = 12 \left(\frac{G}{28.3} \right)$

Rationale

Step 1: we are looking for the weight of the cake in ounces (X), so X must be on the left of the equals sign.

Step 2: we are given the serving size in grams, but we are looking for a weight in ounces, so we need to convert grams to ounces. We are told that grams are converted to ounces by dividing by 28.3, so one serving size in ounces $= \frac{G}{28.3}$

Step 3: we are looking for the weight of a cake providing 12 servings (one for each member of the group), so $\frac{G}{28.3}$ must be multiplied by 12. So the correct formula is $X = 12 \left(\frac{G}{28.3}\right)$.

Answer B is incorrect: $G = \frac{12X}{28.3}$. This is incorrect as it has the G on the left side but it is not grams that are being calculated. We do not need to check the remainder of the equation.

Answer C is incorrect: $G = \frac{12}{28.3X}$. Again this is not correct as it has the G on the left side so we do not have to check the remainder of the equation.

Answer D is incorrect: $X = 28.3 \left(\frac{G}{12}\right)$. Here the 28.3 and the 12 are the wrong way round as we must divide G by 28.3 and then multiply the result by 12.

Answer E is incorrect: $X = \frac{28.3}{12G}$. This is incorrect as G must be divided by 28.3, and the result must be multiplied by 12 rather than divided by it.

Question 21

Addition and subtraction: rule

Performing addition is one of the simplest numerical tasks – it is a mathematical operation that represents combining collections of objects (in this case numbers) together into a larger collection. It is signified by the plus sign (+). To subtract, take one value from another.

Answer B is correct: £1,587.00.

Rationale

Step 1: identify the costs.

2 couples for 2 nights (Fri–Sat): £229 × 4 = £916

1 single for 2 nights (Fri–Sat) + single occupancy supplement: £229 × 1 + £20 = £249.

1 couple for 1 night (Fri) – lodge room deductions: (£139 × 2) – (£5 × 2) = £268.

1 single for 1 night (Fri) + single occupancy supplement – lodge room deductions: (£139 × 1) + £20 – £5 = £154

Step 2: sum the costs: £916 + £249 + £268 + £154 = £1587.

Step 3: the total cost for the golf society is £1,587.00.

Answer A is incorrect: £1607.00. This figure includes a further £20 single supplement for the single person staying two nights whereas the £20 supplement includes both nights.

Answer C is incorrect: £1602.00. This figure does not include the three £5 deductions for the couple and single person staying in the lodge rooms.

Answer D is incorrect: £1507.00. This figure results from using the Mon–Thurs rate of £209 for the two couples staying two nights, and not the Fri–Sat rate of £229.

Answer E is incorrect: £1547.00. This figure results from failing to add on total room supplements of £40 for the two single occupancies.

Question 22

Range: rule

The **range** of a distribution is found by working out the difference between the highest value and the lowest value. The range should always be given as a single value.

Answer C is correct: £160.00.

Rationale

Step 1: the highest value package offered is £289.00.

Step 2: the lowest value package offered is £129.00.

Step 3: the range of prices of the packages is £289.00 – £129.00 = £160.00.

Answer A is incorrect: £129.00. This is the mode of the distribution, i.e. the number that has the highest frequency in the distribution.

Answer B is incorrect: £139.00. Although this is one of the values of the packages, it has no relevance to this question.

Answer D is incorrect: £198.00. This is the mean of the distribution, i.e. the costs of the packages have been summed and divided by the number of values: $\frac{1383}{7}$ = £197.57 (£198 to the nearest whole number).

Answer E is incorrect: £209.00. This is the median of the distribution, i.e. the middle value when all the values are arranged in order.

Question 23

Percentage: rule

A **percentage** is a way of expressing a number as a fraction of 100 (per cent meaning 'per hundred'), denoted using the % sign. Percentages are used to express how large/small one quantity is relevant to another quantity. The first quantity usually represents a part of, or a change in, the second quantity, which should be greater than zero.

Answer A is correct: £281.00.

Rationale

Step 1: 3 nights (Fri–Sun) for 2 couples: £289 × 4 = £1156.

Step 2: special winter deal, 15% reduction: $\frac{1156}{100} \times 85 = £982.60$.

Step 3: spa package for 2 couples: £75 × 2 = £150.

Step 4: special winter deal, 5% reduction = $\frac{150}{100} \times 95 = £142.50$.

Step 5: total cost for 2 couples, with reductions = £1,125.10.

Step 6: total cost per person = $\frac{1125.10}{4}$ = £281.275, or £281.00 to the nearest whole number.

Answer B is incorrect: £283.00. This is the answer where the spa package has not been discounted by 5% = £283.15; i.e. £283.00 to the nearest whole number.

Answer C is incorrect: £246.00. This is the answer where only the 15% reduction on the golf package has been used and no account has been taken of the spa package = £245.65; i.e. £246.00 to the nearest whole number.

Answer D is incorrect: £317.00. This is the answer where the cost of the spa package has been taken as £75 per person discounted at 5% = £316.90; i.e. £317.00 to the nearest whole number.

Answer E is incorrect: £327.00. This is the answer where no discounts have been calculated for either the golf or spa = £326.50; i.e. £327.00 to the nearest whole number.

Question 24

Addition and subtraction: rule

Performing addition is one of the simplest numerical tasks – it is a mathematical operation that represents combining collections of objects (in this case numbers) together into a larger collection. It is signified by the plus sign (+). To subtract, take one value from another.

Answer D is correct: £60.25.

Rationale

Step 1: woman A has three treatments, none of which is marked with an asterisk so she gets three treatments for the price of two i.e. £37.95 × two = £75.90.

Step 2: woman B has three treatments but one of these (reiki) is not part of the 3-for-2 offer, therefore the cost of her treatments is £37.95 × 3 = £113.85.

Step 3: total cost of treatments for the two women is £75.90 + £113.85 = £189.75.

Step 4: the amount of money the woman paying has left is £250.00 – £189.75 = £60.25.

Answer A is incorrect: £174.10. To arrive at this answer, only the costs relating to woman A (£75.90) have been deducted, i.e. £250.00 – £75.90 = £174.10.

Answer B is incorrect: £136.15. To arrive at this answer, only the costs relating to woman B (£113.85) have been deducted, i.e. £250.00 – £113.85 = £136.15.

Answer C is incorrect: £98.20. To arrive at this answer, the costs of treatments for both women have been calculated on a 3-for-2 basis (£151.80) and then deducted, i.e. £250.00 – £151.80 = £98.20.

Answer E is incorrect: £22.30. To arrive at this answer, no 3-for-2 discount has been taken into account and the full cost of six treatments used (£227.70) and then deducted, i.e. £250.00 – £227.70 = £22.30.

Question 25

Percentages (fraction): rule
To change a **fraction** to a **percentage** multiply by 100.

Answer D is correct: 58%.

Rationale
Step 1: find the number of competitors that had a failed vault when the bar was set at 4.6 metres; this is 7.

Step 2: the fraction of competitors who had a failed vault is therefore $\frac{7}{12}$ where 12 is the number of competitors.

Step 3: to change the fraction to a percentage, multiply by 100%, i.e. $\frac{7}{12} \times 100\% = 58.33\%$.

Step 4: therefore 58% of competitors, to the nearest whole number, had a failed vault when the bar was set at 4.6 metres.

Answer A is incorrect: 33%. To arrive at this answer, the number of competitors who had a failed vault at 4.6 metres would need to be 4, i.e. $\frac{4}{12} \times 100\% = 33.33\%$, or 33% to the nearest whole number.

Answer B is incorrect: 42%. To arrive at this answer, the number of competitors who had a failed vault at 4.6 metres would need to be 5, i.e. $\frac{5}{12} \times 100\% = 41.66\%$, or 42% to the nearest whole number.

Answer C is incorrect: 50%. To arrive at this answer, the number of competitors who had a failed vault at 4.6 metres would need to be 6, i.e. $\frac{6}{12} \times 100\% = 50\%$.

Answer E is incorrect: 67%. To arrive at this answer, the number of competitors who had a failed vault at 4.6 metres would need to be 8, i.e. $\frac{8}{12} \times 100\% = 66.66\%$, or 67% to the nearest whole number.

Question 26

Fractions: rule

To find one number as a **fraction** of another, you write the numbers as a fraction, with the first number on the top and the second number on the bottom. The top line of a fraction is called the numerator and the bottom line of a fraction is called the denominator.

Answer E is correct: $\frac{3}{10}$

Rationale

Step 1: the number of failed vaults = 15 (numerator).

Step 2: the total number of vaults = 50 (denominator).

Step 3: write the number as a fraction, i.e. $\frac{15}{50}$. Both the numerator and denominator are divisible by 5, so the fraction can be simplified to $\frac{3}{10}$.

Step 4: the number of failed vaults that occurred compared to the total number of vaults, expressed as a fraction, is $\frac{3}{10}$.

Answer A is incorrect: $\frac{1}{4}$. For this answer to be correct, the number of failed vaults would need to be 12 and the successful vaults 48, i.e. $\frac{12}{48} = \frac{1}{4}$.

Answer B is incorrect: $\frac{1}{3}$. For this answer to be correct, the number of failed vaults would need to be 16 and the successful vaults 48, i.e. $\frac{16}{48} = \frac{1}{3}$.

Answer C is incorrect: $\frac{1}{2}$. For this answer to be correct, the number of failed vaults would need to be 25 and the successful vaults 50, i.e. $\frac{25}{50} = \frac{1}{2}$.

Answer D is incorrect: $\frac{2}{9}$. For this answer to be correct, the number of failed vaults would need to be 12 and the successful vaults 54, i.e. $\frac{12}{54} = \frac{2}{9}$.

Question 27

Ratios: rule

A **ratio** allows one quantity to be compared to another quantity. Any two numbers can be compared by writing them alongside each other with the numbers being separated by a ratio sign (:).

Answer B is correct: 1:3.

Rationale

Step 1: three competitors failed more than one vault when the bar was set at 5.2 metres and a total of nine competitors remained in the competition.

Step 2: write these figures separated by the ratio sign, i.e. 3:9.

Step 3: cancel these numbers if possible; on this occasion both numbers are divisible by 3, to give a ratio of 1:3.

Answer A is incorrect: 1:2. This answer results from counting all those competitors failing the vault at this height (i.e. 6) and comparing this to all those in the competition, ignoring those eliminated (12), giving a ratio of 6:12; both numbers are divisible by 6, which leaves 1:2.

Answer C is incorrect: 1:4. This answer results from comparing the number of competitors with more than one failed vault with all those in the competition, i.e. 3:12; both numbers are divisible by 3, giving a ratio of 1:4.

Answer D is incorrect: 2:3. As in answer A above, this results from counting 6 competitors with a failed vault, but this time comparing with the number of competitors remaining, i.e. 6:9; both numbers are divisible by 3, giving a ratio of 2:3.

Answer E is incorrect: 3:4. This answer results from comparing the number of competitors remaining with the original number in the competition, i.e. 9:12; both numbers are divisible by 3, giving a ratio of 3:4.

Question 28

Mean: rule
The mean or average of a distribution is found by summing the values of the distribution and dividing by the number of values.

Answer D is correct: 5.3 metres.

Rationale
Step 1: identify from the chart the greatest height that each competitor successfully vaulted: 4.4, 4.6, 4.8, 5.2, 5.2, 5.4, 5.4, 5.6, 5.6, 5.8, 5.8, 6.0.

Step 2: sum the heights identified, i.e. 4.4 + 4.6 + 4.8 + 5.2 + 5.2 + 5.4 + 5.4 + 5.6 + 5.6 + 5.8 + 5.8 + 6.0 = 63.8.

Step 3: to obtain the average, divide the sum of the numbers by the number of competitors, i.e. $\frac{63.8}{12}$ = 5.3 metres, to one decimal place.

Answer A is incorrect: 5.0 metres. This would be the mean if the sum of the values was 60, i.e. $\frac{60}{12}$ = 5.0 metres.

Answer B is incorrect: 5.1 metres. This would be the mean if the sum of the values was 61.4, i.e. $\frac{61.4}{12}$ = 5.1 metres.

Answer C is incorrect: 5.2 metres. This would be the mean if the sum of the values was 62.4, i.e. $\frac{62.4}{12}$ = 5.2 metres.

Answer E is incorrect: 5.4 metres. This would be the mean if the sum of the values was 64.9, i.e. $\frac{64.9}{12}$ = 5.4 metres.

Question 29

Multi-stage calculations: rule

This question contains **addition**, **subtraction**, **multiplication** and **percentages**.

Answer D is correct: Pure Media.

Rationale

Step 1: calculate the cost of each broadband provider to ascertain the cheapest.

Step 2: Pure Media: £40.00 off; 6 months at £12.00 = £72.00 − £40.00 = £32.00.

Answer A is incorrect: Chat-Chat. 40% reduction for 6 months; 60% of £12.00 = $\frac{60}{100}$ × 12 = £7.20 x 6 months = £43.20.

Answer B is incorrect: Yellow. 3 months free = 3 months at £12.50 = £37.50.

Answer C is incorrect: E20. No special offers; 6 months at £7.50 = £45.00.

Answer E is incorrect: DTT. £1.00 for the first 3 months = £3.00; 3 months at £15.00 = £45.00 + £3.00 = £48.00.

Question 30

Mean: rule

The **mean** (or arithmetic mean) of a distribution is found by summing the values of the distribution and dividing by the number of values.

Answer B is correct: The mean average monthly contract cost of the five providers to the nearest £ is £12.00.

Rationale

Step 1: the mean monthly contract cost is the sum of the values divided by the number of values.

Step 2: the sum of the values is 59 and the number of values is 5. Therefore $\frac{59}{5}$ = 11.8 which to the nearest £ is £12.00.

Answer A is incorrect: Only providers with unlimited downloads have 24MB speed. Yellow and Pure Media are the only two providers with unlimited downloads and 24MB speed but E20 with 40GB downloads also has 24MB speed.

Answer C is incorrect: There is a 50% cost difference in the providers who only offer an 18 months contract. The two providers are E20 at £7.50 and DTT at £15.00; the cost difference is actually 100%.

Answer D is incorrect: The monthly contract cost of providers with 20GB downloads is less than those having 40GB downloads. Chat-Chat has 20GB downloads and costs £12 per month. However, E20 with 40GB downloads only costs £7.50 per month.

Answer E is incorrect: Providers who offer 20MB speeds require an 18 months contract. DTT offers 20MB speeds and requires an 18 months contract. However, Chat-Chat who also offers 20MB speeds only requires a 12 months contract.

Question 31

Percentage change: rule

To work out the **percentage change**, work out the increase or decrease and divide it by the original amount, then multiply by 100. Percentage change = (change ÷ original amount) × 100, where the change may be an increase, decrease, profit, loss, error, etc.

Answer C is correct: 69%.

Rationale

Step 1: gather all the relevant information required for the calculations. E20 has no special offers and costs £7.50 per month for 18 months; DTT has a special offer of £1.00 per month for the first 3 months and then £15.00 per month for 15 months.

Step 2: calculate the cost for 18 months for E20; £7.50 per month for 18 months = £135.00.

Step 3: calculate the cost for 18 months for DTT; £1.00 per month for the first 3 months = £3 + 15 months at £15.00 = £228.00.

Step 4: difference in cost = £228.00 − £135.00 = £93.00.

Step 5: percentage difference (increase ÷ original amount) x 100 = $\frac{93}{135}$ x 100 = 68.88 = 69% (to the nearest whole number).

Answer A is incorrect: 47%. A 47% increase can quickly be discounted as £93.00 is well over 50% of the £135.

Answer B is incorrect: 60%. You would have to do the full calculations to disregard this option.

Answer D is incorrect: 77%. You would have to do the full calculations to disregard this option.

Answer E is incorrect: 85%. An 85% increase can quickly be discounted as £93.00 could not be over 80% of £135.00.

Question 32

Multi-stage calculations: rule

This question contains **addition**, **subtraction** and **multiplication**.

Answer A is correct: £104.00.

Rationale

Step 1: identify the broadband providers that fit the criteria 'minimum 24MB speed, 40GB for downloads and a 12 months contract'.

Step 2: only Yellow and Pure Media fit the criteria.

Step 3: the cheapest is Pure Media; £40.00 off; 12 months at £12.00 = £144.00 − £40.00 = £104.00.

Answer B is incorrect: £112.50. This is the cost of Yellow. First 3 months free; 9 months at £12.50 = £112.50.

Answer C is incorrect: £138.00. This is the cost of DTT; − £1.00 a month for first 3 months = £3.00; 9 months at £15.00 = £135.00 + 3 = £138.00. Also DTT does not meet the criteria as it has an 18 months contract where 12 months was specified.

Answer D is incorrect: £144.00. This is the cost of Pure Media over 12 months without taking account of the £40.00 off special offer; 12 months at £12.00 = £144.00.

Answer E is incorrect: £150.00. This is the cost of Yellow over 12 months without taking account of the first 3 months being free; 12 months at £12.50 = £150.00.

Question 33

Multi-stage calculations and conversion: rule

This question contains multiplication, addition and division. The equation for **converting** knots to miles per hour is 1 knot = 1.15 mph.

Answer D is correct: 0400 hours, Thursday 4 March.

Rationale

Step 1: convert knots to miles per hour: $15 \times 1.15 = 17.25$ mph.

Step 2: calculate time at sea: $\frac{1138}{17.25} = 65.97$ hours i.e. $\frac{65.97}{24} = 2.748$ days – approximate to 2.75 days = 2 days 18 hours + 1 hour for time difference = 2 days 19 hours.

Step 3: 0900 hours Monday 1 March + 2 days 19 hours = 0400 hours Thursday 4 March.

Answer A is incorrect: 1800 hours, Wednesday 3 March. This answer is random, i.e. it has not been obtained by using any of the figures provided in the question.

Answer B is incorrect: 0200 hours, Thursday 4 March. This answer has in fact deducted one hour for the time difference between Liverpool and Bilbao instead of adding it.

Answer C is incorrect: 0300 hours, Thursday 4 March. This answer has simply failed to add on the extra hour for the time difference between Liverpool and Bilbao.

Answer E is incorrect: 1400 hours, Thursday 4 March. This answer has used knots only in the calculations failing to convert it to miles per hour.

Question 34

Multi-stage calculations and conversion: rule

This question contains multiplication, addition and division. The equation for **converting** knots to kilometres per hour is 1 knot = 1.852 kilometres per hour.

Answer B is correct: 4.5 laps.

Rationale

Step 1: 3 knots for 10 minutes: $3 \times 1.852 = 5.6$ km/h: $\frac{10}{60} \times 5.6 = 0.9$ kilometres.

Step 2: 10 knots for 20 minutes: $10 \times 1.852 = 18.5$ km/h: $\frac{20}{60} \times 18.5 = 6.2$ kilometres.

Step 3: 7 knots for 30 minutes: $7 \times 1.852 = 13.0$ km/h: $\frac{30}{60} \times 13.0 = 6.5$ kilometres.

Step 4: sum number of kilometres: $0.9 + 6.2 + 6.5 = 13.6$ kilometres.

Step 5: divide distance travelled by course size: $\frac{13.6}{3} = 4.5$ laps.

Answer A is incorrect: 3.5 laps. This answer has miscalculated *Step 2* where it has not converted the 10 knots to km/h providing a figure of 3.3 kilometres instead of 6.2 kilometres.

Answer C is incorrect: 6.0 laps. The answer has incorrectly calculated *Step 4* using the figure 5.6 instead of 0.9 from *Step 1* thereby arriving at a sum of 18 kilometres instead of 13.6.

Answer D is incorrect: 6.7 laps. The answer has incorrectly calculated *Step 4* using the figure 13.0 instead of 6.5 from *Step 3* thereby arriving at a sum of 20.1 kilometres instead of 13.6.

Answer E is incorrect: 12.3 laps. This answer has summed the speed in knots, i.e. $3 \times 10 \times 7 = 20$, converted this to kilometres and divided the answer by the length of the course.

Question 35

Percentage change: rule

To work out the **percentage change**, work out the increase or decrease and divide it by the original amount, then multiply by 100. Percentage change = (change ÷ original amount) × 100, where the change may be an increase, decrease, profit, loss, error, etc.

Answer E is correct: 24%.

Rationale

Step 1: distance left to travel: 58% = 768 nm, therefore 100% of journey = $\frac{768}{58}$ × 100 = 1,324 nm.

Step 2: total oil used: $\frac{1,324}{4}$ × 10 = 3,310 litres.

Step 3: oil remaining: 68% of $\frac{7,500}{100}$ × 68 = 5,100 – 3,310 = 1,790 litres.

Step 4: 1,790 litres as a percentage of 7,500 litres: $\frac{1,790}{7,500}$ × 100 = 24%.

Answer A is incorrect: 7%. At *Step 1*, 42% was used in the calculation instead of 58%.

Answer B is incorrect: 14%. At *Step 3*, 58% was used in the calculation instead of 68%.

Answer C is incorrect: 15%. At *Step 1*, 68% was used in the calculation instead of 58%.

Answer D is incorrect: 18%. At *Step 4*, 1,324 nm was used in the calculation instead of 1,790 litres.

Question 36

Multi-stage calculations and conversion: rule

This question contains multiplication, addition and division. The equation for **converting** sterling to euros is £1 = €1.16.

Answer C is correct: €221.13.

Rationale

Step 1: convert 54p to euros = £0.54 x 1.16 = €0.63.

Step 2: 30 return journeys at 140 miles = 4,200 miles.

Step 3: 4,200 miles divided by 5 miles per litre of fuel = $\frac{4200}{5}$ = 840 litres.

Step 4: fuel remaining = 1,200 – 840 = 360 litres.

Step 5: 360 litres @ €0.63 per litre = €226.80.

Step 6: deduct 2.5% = $\frac{226.80}{100}$ × 2.5 = €5.67.

Step 7: the value of the fuel remaining in the tank is €226.80 – €5.67 = €221.13.

Note: The calculations can be done differently to arrive at the correct answer, for example, at *Step 1* the cost in euros of one litre of fuel could be obtained or the conversion to euros could be left until *Step 7*.

Answer A is incorrect: €164.97. This answer has miscalculated *Step 1* in converting pounds to euros. Instead of multiplying, it has divided 54p by €1.16. Therefore at *Step 5* it has multiplied 360 by €0.47 (€169.20) and not €0.63 and then deducted 2.5% to arrive at this answer.

Answer B is incorrect: €169.20. This answer has miscalculated *Step 1* in converting pounds to euros. Instead of multiplying, it has divided 54p by €1.16. Therefore at *Step 5* it has multiplied 360 by €0.47 (€169.20) and not €0.63 and has failed to deduct the 2.5%.

Answer D is incorrect: €226.80. The answer has failed to complete *Step 6*, i.e. it has failed to deduct the 2.5%.

Answer E is incorrect: €232.47. At *Step 6* and *7* this answer has calculated the 2.5% but then added it to the value of the fuel remaining in the tank rather than deducting it.

Chapter 10
The Abstract Reasoning subtest

This chapter will help you to:

- understand the purpose and format of abstract reasoning tests;
- prepare for the Abstract Reasoning subtest using general abstract reasoning questions;
- test your knowledge and understanding of abstract reasoning-type questions;
- identify those abstract reasoning skills where development is required.

Introduction

Pearson VUE describes the purpose of this subtest as follows: 'The Abstract Reasoning subtest assesses candidates' ability to infer relationships from information by convergent and divergent thinking.'

First, we will clarify what is generally meant by convergent and divergent thinking. These styles of thinking, or cognitive styles, were first identified and named by J.P. Guilford in the 1950s and have been extensively researched since. The following is a brief description of the two styles.

Convergent thinking

The problem-solving skills associated with convergent thinking are characterised by the tendency to focus on the one correct, or single best, solution to a problem. Therefore problems that have unique solutions lend themselves well to convergent thinking.

Divergent thinking

The problem-solving skills associated with divergent thinking are characterised by the ability to produce a number of novel ideas that are relevant to a particular problem. Therefore open-ended problems that do not have unique solutions lend themselves well to divergent thinking.

How are convergent and divergent thinking usually measured?

Convergent thinking is usually measured by conventional multiple-choice questions that have unique correct answers (as in the Abstract Reasoning subtest). The measurement of divergent thinking attempts to tap more creative approaches by asking for more solutions to the problem, of which more than one answer could be correct.

The UKCAT claims for the Abstract Reasoning subtest are as follows.

The items include irrelevant and distracting material which can lead the individual to unsatisfactory solutions. The non-critical person may remain satisfied with such solutions. The test therefore measures both an ability to change track, critically evaluate and to generate hypotheses which can be relevant in the development of new ideas and systems.

However, the format of the subtest does appear to be based on convergent thinking as each question has a unique correct answer.

You may be interested to know that research has found that convergers usually specialise in physical sciences, mathematics or classics, hold conventional attitudes and opinions, pursue technical or mechanical interests, and tend to be emotionally inhibited. Divergers, on the other hand, usually specialise in the arts or biology, hold unconventional attitudes and opinions, pursue interests involving interaction with others, and tend to be emotionally uninhibited. It has been suggested that divergent thinking is an essential prerequisite of exceptional intellectual performance. However, candidates for higher education have usually been selected on the basis of exam results, which generally tap convergent thinking, and the UKCAT appears to be the same.

What are abstract reasoning tests?

Abstract reasoning tests purport to measure 'general intelligence' or 'general intellectual reasoning ability'. General intelligence is supposedly our innate capacity to reason as opposed to our socially and educationally developed verbal and numerical reasoning capacity. Some argue that verbal and numerical reasoning tests can probe innate skills (as does the UKCAT), but there is a strong correlation between the results from GCSEs and A-levels with tests of aptitude. The arguments about intelligence theories are vast and, to some extent, have never been resolved. However, increasingly employers and educational institutions are using reasoning tests as selection measures. Therefore we need to attempt to 'level the playing field'.

Abstract reasoning tests attempt to measure how well you can solve problems from basic principles. To answer these types of questions, you need to identify the underlying logic. Abstract reasoning questions are usually presented in sequences of symbols, patterns or shapes arranged in squares or rows. Examples of these types of questions are in the 'Example questions' section of this chapter.

Typically, to answer these types of questions, you have to work through three stages.

Stage one

The identification of the symbols or shapes used and what they have in common. For example, the things to look for will be as follows.

- *Number*: the number of symbols or shapes.
- *Size*: do the shapes or symbols vary in size – small to large?
- *Shape*: various symbols, circles, squares, triangles or other multi-sided or faceted shapes.
- *Characteristics*: curved lines, straight lines, dotted lines, number or type of angles or points, open sides to shapes, divided shapes, shapes that can be drawn with or without removing the pencil from the paper or back tracking (for example, an X or a square).
- *Colour*: colour may be used, but not usually; could be negative to positive (e.g. black to white or vice versa).

Stage two

The identification of the pattern that the symbols or shapes form:

- *Repeating patterns*: the symbols repeated in twos, threes, fours, etc.
- *Rotation*: the symbol or shape rotated clockwise or anti-clockwise.
- *Mirror images*: are the symbols or shapes mirror images (e.g. flipped left to right or top to bottom)?
- *Direction*: do the symbols or shapes move from top left, to top right, to bottom right, to bottom left, or do they move diagonally?

Stage three

Generally, this would be the identification of which symbol(s), shape(s), etc. form the next part of the sequence. In the case of the UKCAT Abstract Reasoning subtest it is the identification of whether the 'test shape' belongs with 'Set A', 'Set B' or 'Neither Set'. Therefore, you will need to use the processes described in stage one and stage two above to determine whether the test shape has the same characteristics as Set A, Set B or Neither Set.

Abstract Reasoning subtest

The Abstract Reasoning subtest is an on-screen test that consists of 65 items associated with 13 pairs of Set A and Set B shapes. Five test shapes are presented with each pair of Set A and Set B shapes and there are three answer options for each test shape: Set A,

Set B or Neither Set. Only ONE of the three answer options is correct. Each test shape is presented with the pair of Set A and Set B shapes on a separate screen with the three answer options below. A period of sixteen minutes is allowed for the test, with one minute for instruction and the remaining fifteen minutes for items.

Before attempting the practice questions based on the approach taken in the UKCAT, you should find it beneficial to work through the following example questions.

The first three examples based on classic abstract reasoning items have just one question. Examples 4 and 5 relate to two sets of shapes (four boxes in each set) but with the same response format of the UKCAT. The final examples (6 and 7) are based on the UKCAT format and will serve as a 'trial run' prior to attempting the abstract reasoning practice test. This staged approach should develop your understanding of how this type of reasoning test is structured and should also develop your confidence and ability when answering the questions.

Sets of shapes and response formats

The sets of shapes are normally regular or irregular shapes and symbols which are usually black and white, but colour may be used. For the purpose of the UKCAT, the two sets of shapes (Set A and Set B) each contain six boxes. Each pair of sets will be followed by five test shapes which have to be matched to the response format of Set A, Set B or Neither Set. The example questions will clarify this.

Example questions

The following three examples require you to select the correct answer from the six options provided.

Example 1

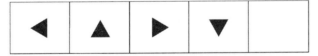

What comes next?

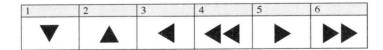

Rationale

Stage 1: the shapes in the question are all single, same-size, black triangles.

Stage 2: the triangles rotate clockwise by 90° each time.

Stage 3: the solution must be a single, black triangle; the triangle must be rotated clockwise by a further 90°.

Distracters: options 1, 2 and 5 could be considered but can be eliminated, as there is not a logical pattern.

Irrelevant: options 4 and 6 can be eliminated immediately as logic points to a single black triangle.

The answer to Example 1 is 3. The triangle will be back in the original position, as at the start of the sequence.

Example 2

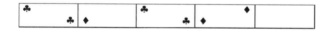

What comes next?

1	2	3	4	5	6
♣ ♣	♦ ♦	♦ ♦	♣	♣ ♣ ♣	♣ ♣

Rationale

Stage 1: the shapes in the question are all black, same-size clubs or diamonds; there are three groups of two shapes and one single shape.

Stage 2: the shapes are sequenced 2, 1, 2 and 2; the only repeat is the alternating two clubs in the same position.

Stage 3: the solution must be two clubs.

Distracters: options 1, 5 and 6 could be considered but can be eliminated, as there is no logical pattern.

Irrelevant: options 2 and 3 are diamonds and can be eliminated immediately as logic points to clubs.

The answer to Example 2 is 4. The two clubs are in the same position.

Example 3

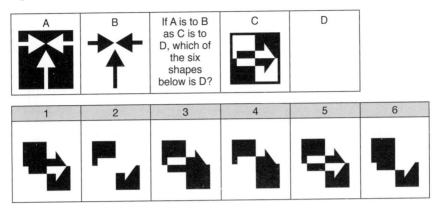

Rationale

Stage 1: the shapes in boxes A and B of the question are the same but B is the negative of A (e.g. white to black and black to white); the shape in box C is different from A and B.

Stage 2: the shape in box C must relate to box D using the same criteria as the relationship between A and B.

Stage 3: the solution must be a negative of C.

Distracters: all the other options are distracters but can be easily discounted when examined for change from black to white and vice versa.

Irrelevant: all options could have been relevant on the basis of shape.

The answer to Example 3 is 5. This is the negative of item C.

The following two examples use a format very similar to the UKCAT in that you have to match a test shape to Set A, Set B or Neither Set. However, in this staged approach we are using only four boxes in Set A and B as opposed to the six used in the UKCAT. The key point is, first, to determine what distinguishes each set to arrive at the rationale. Answering the associated questions should then be a relatively quick process as the test shapes will contain the key characteristics identified as belonging to Set A, Set B or Neither Set.

Examples 4 and 5

Set A

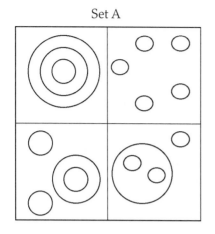

Set B

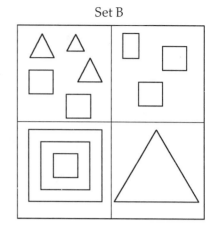

Example 4 Test Shape

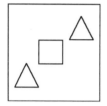

Example 5 Test Shape

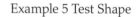
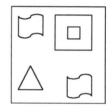

Rationale

Stage 1: the shapes in Set A are all circles, the shapes in Set B are triangles and/or squares; the size and number of the shapes vary in both sets; the shapes are all white in both sets; shapes can be within others in both sets; the shapes in Set A are all circular (curved lines), the shapes in Set B have straight lines only.

Stage 2: both sets contain no logical repeats, rotations, mirror images or direction changes.

Stage 3: therefore, the solution must be the Stage 1 characteristic of shapes with curved lines in Set A and shapes with straight lines in Set B. Any test shape containing both will belong with Neither Set.

Distracters: shapes, numbers of shapes and position of shapes (including shapes within others).

Irrelevant: two different shapes in Set B.

The answer to Example 4 is Set B. The test shape belongs to Set B as all the shapes have straight lines.

The answer to Example 5 is Neither Set. The test shape belongs to Neither Set as two of the shapes have both straight and curved lines.

The following examples are based on the UKCAT format.

Examples 6 and 7

Set A

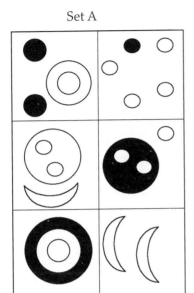

Set B

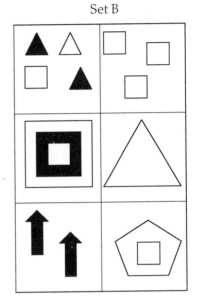

Example 6 Test Shape

Example 7 Test Shape

Rationale

Stage 1: the shapes in Set A include circles, ovals and crescents; the shapes in Set B include triangles, squares, rectangles and arrows; the size and number of the shapes vary in both sets; the shapes are white, black or black and white in both sets; shapes can be within others in both sets; the shapes in Set A all have curved lines, the shapes in Set B all have straight lines.

Stage 2: both sets contain no logical repeats, rotations, mirror images or direction changes.

Stage 3: therefore, the solution must be the Stage 1 characteristic of shapes with curved lines in Set A and shapes with straight lines in Set B. Any test shape containing both will belong with Neither Set.

Distracters: shapes, numbers of shapes, position of shapes and shapes within others.

Irrelevant: different shapes in both sets and use of black.

The answer to Example 6 is Neither Set. The test shape belongs to Neither Set as the shapes have both straight and curved lines.

The answer to Example 7 is Set B. The test shape belongs to Set B as the shapes all have straight lines.

Abstract Reasoning practice subtest

The Abstract Reasoning practice subtest provided below is a full test comprising 65 items associated with 13 pairs of Set A and Set B shapes. These questions do not replicate those used in the UKCAT but are of the same format. The shapes in Set A are related in some way, as are the shapes in Set B, but the sets are not related to each other. Following each pair of sets there are five test shapes (questions). Examine Set A and Set B using the stages described in the introductory section, and decide whether each individual test shape belongs to Set A, Set B or Neither Set.

If you want to simulate 'test conditions', you are advised to use rough paper to mark down your choice for each of the questions (i.e. Set A, Set B or Neither Set). A period of 16 minutes is allowed for the subtest, with one minute for administration and the remaining 15 minutes to answer the questions.

The correct answer and rationale to each of the questions are produced in the section following the practice subtest.

Questions 1 to 5

Set A

Set B

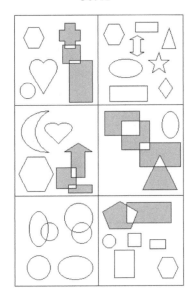
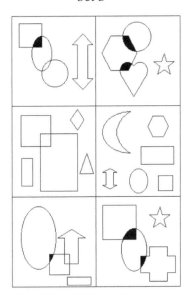

Test Shapes

Question 1   Question 2   Question 3   Question 4   Question 5

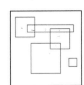

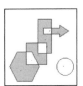

Questions 6 to 10

Set A   Set B

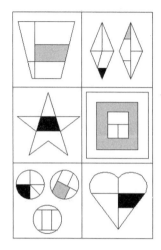   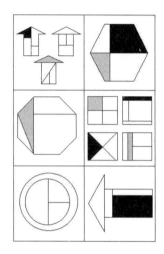

Test Shapes

Question 6   Question 7   Question 8   Question 9   Question 10

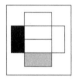

Questions 11 to 15

Set A

Set B

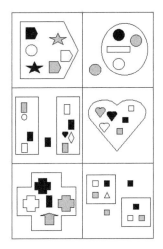

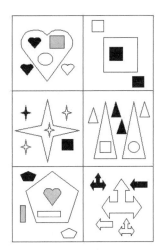

Test Shapes

Question 11   Question 12   Question 13   Question 14   Question 15

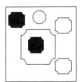 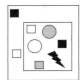 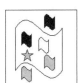

Questions 16 to 20

Set A

Set B

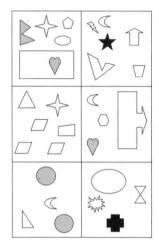
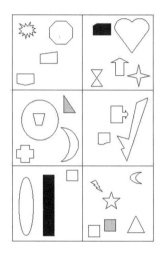

Test Shapes

Question 16   Question 17   Question 18   Question 19   Question 20

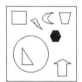

Questions 21 to 25

Set A

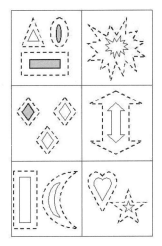

Set B

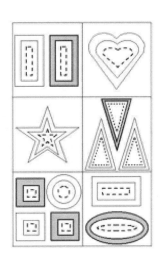

Test Shapes

Question 21   Question 22   Question 23   Question 24   Question 25

 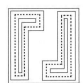 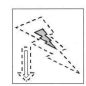 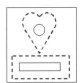

Questions 26 to 30

Set A

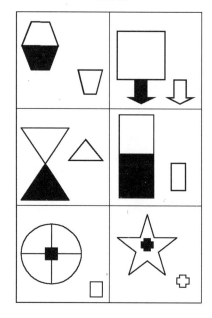

Set B

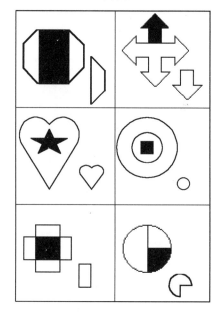

Test Shapes

Question 26	Question 27	Question 28	Question 29	Question 30

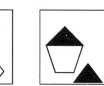
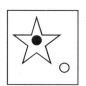

Questions 31 to 35

Set A

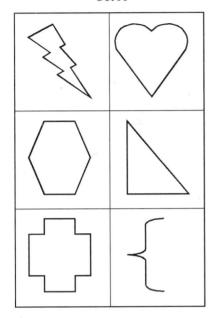

Set B

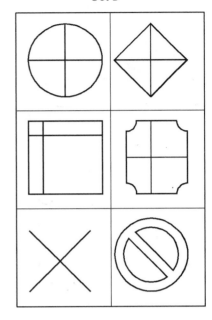

Test Shapes

Question 31   Question 32   Question 33   Question 34   Question 35

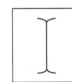 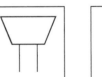 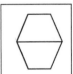

Questions 36 to 40

Set A   Set B

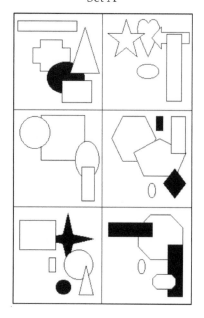   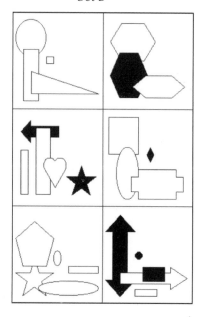

Test Shapes

Question 36   Question 37   Question 38   Question 39   Question 40

        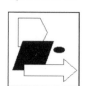

Questions 41 to 45

Set A

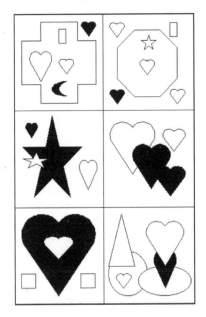

Set B

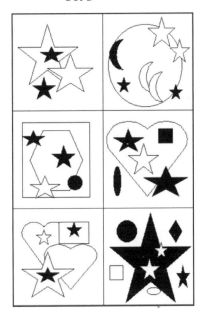

Test Shapes

Question 41   Question 42   Question 43   Question 44   Question 45

 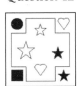 

Questions 46 to 50

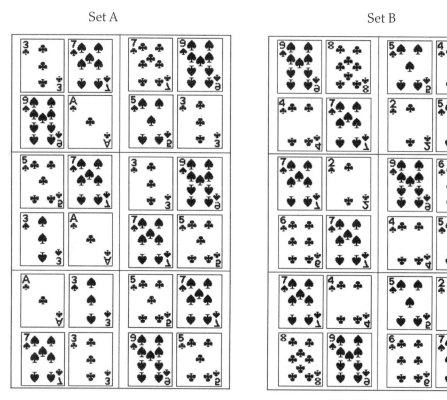

Set A   Set B

Test Shapes

Question 46   Question 47   Question 48   Question 49   Question 50

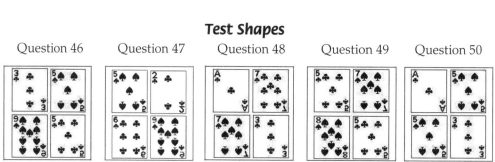

Questions 51 to 55

Set A

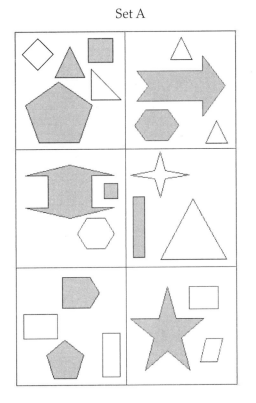

Set B

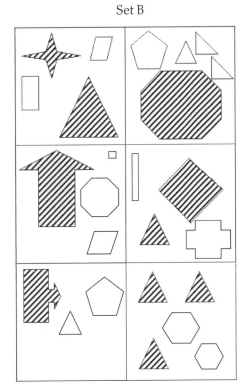

Test Shapes

Question 51   Question 52   Question 53   Question 54   Question 55

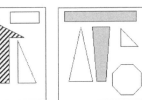   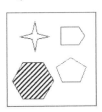   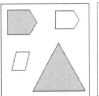   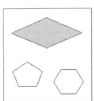

Questions 56 to 60

Set A

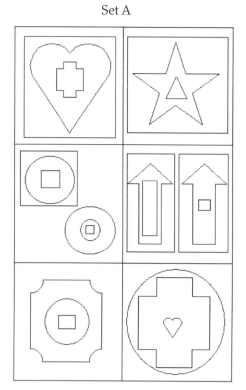

Set B

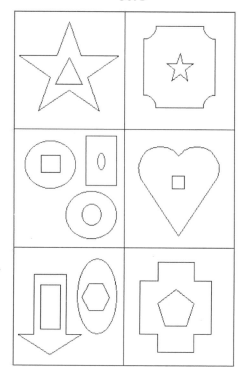

Test Shapes

Question 56

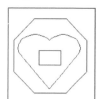

Question 57

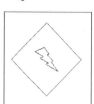

Question 58

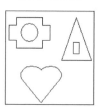

Question 59

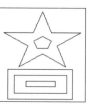

Question 60

Questions 61 to 65

Set A · Set B

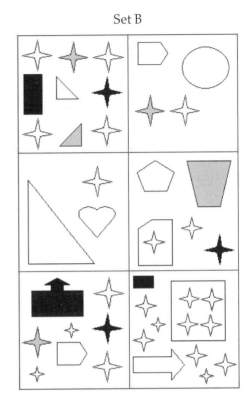

Test Shapes

Question 61 · Question 62 · Question 63 · Question 64 · Question 65

Abstract Reasoning practice subtest: answers

Question number	Correct response	Question number	Correct response
1	Neither Set	34	Set B
2	Set B	35	Set A
3	Neither Set	36	Set B
4	Neither Set	37	Neither Set
5	Set A	38	Set B
6	Neither Set	39	Set A
7	Set B	40	Neither Set
8	Neither Set	41	Neither Set
9	Neither Set	42	Set B
10	Set A	43	Neither Set
11	Set B	44	Set B
12	Neither Set	45	Set A
13	Set B	46	Set A
14	Set A	47	Set B
15	Neither Set	48	Neither Set
16	Set B	49	Neither Set
17	Neither Set	50	Set A
18	Set B	51	Neither Set
19	Set A	52	Neither Set
20	Neither Set	53	Set B
21	Set B	54	Set A
22	Neither Set	55	Set A
23	Set B	56	Set A
24	Set A	57	Set B
25	Neither Set	58	Neither Set
26	Neither Set	59	Neither Set
27	Set B	60	Set A
28	Set A	61	Set B
29	Neither Set	62	Neither Set
30	Set A	63	Set A
31	Set A	64	Set B
32	Set B	65	Set A
33	Set A		

Abstract Reasoning practice subtest: explanation of answers

Questions 1 to 5

Rationale

Stage 1: the shapes in Set A include a cross, diamond, star, crescent and a pentagon, and hexagons, hearts, squares, rectangles, circles, arrows, triangles and ovals; the shapes in Set B include a heart, hexagon, diamond, triangle, crescent and a cross, and squares, ovals, circles, arrows, stars and rectangles; the sizes of the shapes differ in both sets; the numbers of the different shapes vary in both sets; the shapes are white and grey in Set A and white and black in Set B but there is more grey in Set A than black in Set B.

Stage 2: both sets contain no rotations, mirror images or direction changes; however, both sets contain a logical repeat: in Set A all the boxes contain shapes with eight enclosed areas (including the overlaps); if straight-sided shapes overlap then the remainder of the shape is grey. In Set B all the boxes contain shapes with six enclosed areas (including the overlaps); if a shape with a curved side overlaps one with a straight side then the overlap is black.

Stage 3: therefore, the solution must lie in the *Stage 2* characteristic of each box in Set A containing shapes with eight enclosed areas where the remaining part of overlapping straight-sided shapes is grey, and each box in Set B containing shapes with six enclosed areas where the overlap between a curved-sided shape and a straight-sided shape is black. Any test shape not meeting these criteria belongs to Neither Set.

Distracters: shapes, numbers of shapes, size of shapes, position of shapes and boxes containing no shading.

Irrelevant: different shapes in both sets.

Answer to question 1 is Neither Set: the test shape belongs to Neither Set as the remaining parts of the overlapping straight-sided shapes need to be grey to meet the Set A criteria, and there are too many enclosed areas for Set B.

Answer to question 2 is Set B: the test shape belongs to Set B as there are six enclosed areas and no overlaps between curved-sided and straight-sided shapes.

Answer to question 3 is Neither Set: the test shape belongs to Neither Set as the remaining parts of the overlapping straight-sided shapes need to be grey to meet the Set A criteria, and there are too many enclosed areas for Set B.

Answer to question 4 is Neither Set: the test shape belongs to Neither Set as the overlap between the square and the circle should be black in order to belong to Set B.

Answer to question 5 is Set A: the test shape belongs to Set A as there are eight enclosed areas and the remaining parts of the overlapping straight-sided shapes are grey.

Questions 6 to 10

Rationale

Stage 1: the shapes in Set A include a rhomboid, star and a heart, and diamonds, squares and circles; the shapes in Set B include a hexagon and an octagon, and arrows, squares and circles; the sizes of the shapes differ in both sets; the number of shapes vary in both sets; the shapes are white, grey and black in both sets; the individual shapes within the boxes are divided into five in Set A and into four in Set B.

Stage 2: both sets contain no rotations, mirror images or direction changes.

Stage 3: therefore, the solution must be the *Stage 1* characteristic of individual shapes being divided into five and four in Set A and Set B, respectively. Any test shape not meeting the criteria belongs to Neither Set.

Distracters: shapes, numbers of shapes, size of shapes, position of shapes, black and grey shading and shapes within shapes.

Irrelevant: different shapes in both sets.

Answer to question 6 is Neither Set: the test shape belongs to Neither Set as the shape has been divided into six.

Answer to question 7 is Set B: the test shape belongs to Set B as the shapes have been divided into four.

Answer to question 8 is Neither Set: the test shape belongs to Neither Set as one of the shapes has been divided into five and the other four, therefore this test shape has the characteristics of both sets.

Answer to question 9 is Neither Set: the test shape belongs to Neither Set as it has only been divided into three.

Answer to question 10 is Set A: the test shape belongs to Set A as the shape has been divided into five.

Questions 11 to 15

Rationale

Stage 1: the shapes in Set A include a diamond and a triangle, and arrows, stars, circles, rectangles, hearts, squares and crosses; the shapes in Set B include hearts, squares, circles, stars, triangles, pentagons, rectangles and arrows; the sizes of the shapes differ in both sets; the number of shapes vary in both sets; the shapes are white, grey and black in both sets; the shapes have curved and straight lines in both sets.

Stage 2: both sets contain no rotations, mirror images or direction changes; there is a logical repeat in each set: the larger outline shapes in Set A are reflected three times as smaller images within the shape and are shaded white, grey and black; the larger outline shapes in Set B are reflected at least twice as smaller images on the outside of the shape and at least one must be white and one black.

Stage 3: therefore, the solution must be the Stage 2 characteristic of the large shape being reflected as three smaller white, grey and black images within the shape in Set A and the large shape being reflected as two smaller black and white images on the outside of the shape in Set B. Any test shape not meeting the criteria belongs to Neither Set.

Distracters: smaller shapes outside larger shapes in Set A; more than two smaller shapes outside larger shapes in Set B; smaller shapes within larger shapes in Set B and number of shapes.

Irrelevant: different shapes in both sets.

Answer to question 11 is Set B: the test shape belongs to Set B as the large shape is reflected as both a black and white smaller image on the outside of the shape. The additional images outside and within the shape are distracters.

Answer to question 12 is Neither Set: the test shape belongs to Neither Set as the shape is reflected as three smaller white, grey and black images within the shape and is also reflected by a smaller black and white image on the outside of the shape, therefore it has the characteristics of both sets.

Answer to question 13 is Set B: the test shape belongs to Set B as the large shape is reflected as both a black and white smaller image on the outside of the shape.

Answer to question 14 is Set A: the test shape belongs to Set A as the large shape is reflected as three smaller white, grey and black images within the shape. The additional images outside the shape are distracters and are incorrectly coloured for Set B.

Answer to question 15 is Neither Set: the test shape belongs to Neither Set as the larger shape is not repeated against the criteria for either Set A or Set B in terms of shading.

Questions 16 to 20

Rationale

Stage 1: the shapes in Set A include a rectangle, pentagon, rhomboid and a hexagon, and stars, ovals, irregular shapes, hearts, parallelograms, moons, arrows, triangles and circles; the shapes in Set B include an octagon, heart, circle, rhomboid, cross, oval and a rectangle, and irregular shapes, arrows, stars, triangles, moons and squares; the sizes of the shapes differ in both sets; the number of shapes vary in both sets; the shapes are white, grey and black in both sets; the shapes have curved and straight lines in both sets; the shapes in Set A contain one shape which has at least one right angle; the shapes in Set B contain two shapes which have at least one right angle each.

Stage 2: both sets contain no rotations, mirror images or direction changes.

Stage 3: therefore, the solution must be the Stage 1 characteristic of shapes that contain one shape which has at least one right angle in Set A and shapes that contain two shapes which have at least one right angle each in Set B. Any test shape not meeting the criteria belongs to Neither Set.

Distracters: shapes, numbers and size of shapes, shapes within others, duplicate shapes, grey and black shading and the position of shapes.

Irrelevant: the use of other angles.

Answer to question 16 is Set B: the test shape belongs to Set B as it contains two shapes which have at least one right angle each and any shading is a distracter.

Answer to question 17 is Neither Set: the test shape belongs to Neither Set as it contains three shapes which have at least one right angle and this does not meet the criteria for either Set A or Set B.

Answer to question 18 is Set B: the test shape belongs to Set B as it contains two shapes which have at least one right angle each and any shading or shapes within others are distracters.

Answer to question 19 is Set A: the test shape belongs to Set A as it contains one shape which has at least one right angle.

Answer to question 20 is Neither Set: the test shape belongs to Neither Set as it does not contain any shapes with right angles.

Questions 21 to 25

Rationale

Stage 1: the shapes in Set A include triangles, ovals, rectangles, irregular shapes, diamonds, arrows, moons, hearts and stars; the shapes in Set B include rectangles, hearts, stars, triangles, squares, circles and ovals; the sizes of the shapes differ in both sets; the number of shapes vary in both sets; the shapes are white, grey and black in both sets; the shapes have curved and straight lines in both sets; the outlines of all the shapes in Set A are broken and the shape is reflected within with a solid outline, and the outlines of Set B are solid with the shape reflected within twice, the inner of which has a broken outline.

Stage 2: both sets contain no rotations, mirror images or direction changes.

Stage 3: therefore, the solution must be the Stage 1 characteristic of shapes with broken outlines with the shape reflected within with a solid outline in Set A; and shapes with solid outlines with the shape reflected twice within, the inner of which has a broken outline, in Set B. Any test shape not meeting the criteria belongs to Neither Set.

Distracters: shapes, numbers of shapes, size of shapes, position of shapes and shading.

Irrelevant: different shapes in both sets.

Answer to question 21 is Set B: the test shape belongs to Set B as the shape has a solid outline with the shape reflected twice within, the inner of which has a broken outline.

Answer to question 22 is Neither Set: the test shape belongs to Neither Set as the shape has a solid outline with the shape reflected twice within; however, the middle shape has a broken line which would need to be the inner shape if it was to belong to Set B.

Answer to question 23 is Set B: the test shape belongs to Set B as the shape has a solid outline with the shape reflected twice within, the inner of which has a broken outline. The number of shapes is a distracter.

Answer to question 24 is Set A: the test shape belongs to Set A as the shape has a broken outline with the shape reflected within with a solid outline.

Answer to question 25 is Neither Set: the test shape belongs to Neither Set as the shape has a circle instead of a solid outlined heart inside the broken outlined heart, therefore it does not have the correct characteristics for Set A.

Questions 26 to 30

Rationale

Stage 1: the shapes in Set A include a hexagon, trapezium, circle and a star, and squares, arrows, triangles, rectangles and crosses; the shapes in Set B include an octagon, trapezium, star and three quarters of a circle, and rectangles, arrows, hearts, circles and squares; the sizes and numbers of the shapes vary in both sets; the shapes are white, black or black and white in both sets; shapes can be within others in both sets.

Stage 2: both sets contain no rotations, mirror images or direction changes; both sets contain logical repeats: in Set A the black part of the large shape is reflected separately as a white shape which may differ in size; in Set B the separate shape does not reflect the black part of the large shape but it is still white.

Stage 3: therefore, the solution must be the *Stage 2* characteristic of the black part of the larger shape being reflected as a separate white shape in Set A and the black part of the larger shape not being reflected in the smaller white shape in Set B. Any test shape not meeting the criteria belongs to Neither Set.

Distracters: shapes, numbers of shapes, position of shapes, shapes within others and the repeat of part of the shapes in Set B.

Irrelevant: differing shapes in both sets.

Answer to question 26 is Neither Set: the test shape belongs to Neither Set as there is not a smaller white shape.

Answer to question 27 is Set B: the test shape belongs to Set B as the black rectangular part of the large shape is not reflected in the smaller white shape.

Answer to question 28 is Set A: the test shape belongs to Set A as the black arrow within the larger shape is reflected in the smaller white shape.

Answer to question 29 is Neither Set: the test shape belongs to Neither Set as the black triangle from the larger shape is reflected as a smaller black image, not white.

Answer to question 30 is Set A: the test shape belongs to Set A as the black circle within the star is reflected in the smaller white shape.

Questions 31 to 35

Rationale

Stage 1: the shapes and symbols in Set A include a lightning flash, heart, hexagon, triangle, cross and a bracket; the shapes and symbols in Set B include a circle, diamond, square, plaque, 'X' and a 'no entry' symbol; the sizes and numbers of the shapes are equal in both sets; the shapes are white or lines only in both sets; the shapes in Set A can all be drawn without lifting the pen or pencil off the paper; the shapes in Set B have intersecting lines or lines within, which means they cannot be drawn without back-tracking or lifting the pen or pencil off the paper.

Stage 2: both sets contain no logical repeats, rotations, mirror images or direction changes.

Stage 3: therefore, the solution must be the *Stage 1* characteristic of shapes that can be drawn without lifting the pen or pencil off the paper, as in Set A; or shapes that cannot be drawn without back-tracking or lifting the pen or pencil off the paper, as in Set B. Therefore, by definition, all test shapes will meet the criteria for either Set A or Set B.

Distracters: shapes, and single intersecting lines when within shapes as in question 35.

Irrelevant: differing shapes in both sets.

Answer to question 31 is Set A: the test shape belongs to Set A as it can be drawn from any point without lifting the pen or pencil off the paper.

Answer to question 32 is Set B: the test shape belongs to Set B as the two adjoining brackets cannot be drawn from any point without lifting the pen or pencil off the paper.

Answer to question 33 is Set A: the test shape belongs to Set A as it can be drawn from any point without lifting the pen or pencil off the paper.

Answer to question 34 is Set B: the test shape belongs to Set B as the addition of two lines (or legs) to the trapezium means it cannot be drawn from any point without lifting the pen or pencil off the paper.

Answer to question 35 is Set A: the test shape belongs to Set A as it can be drawn without lifting the pen or pencil off the paper, provided you start from either end of the middle or intersecting line.

Questions 36 to 40

Rationale

Stage 1: the shapes in Set A include a cross, heart, arrow, hexagon, pentagon and a diamond, and rectangles, triangles, ovals, squares, stars, circles and octagons; the shapes in Set B include a triangle, heart, diamond, cross, square, circle and a pentagon, and rectangles, hexagons, arrows, stars and ovals; the sizes of the shapes differ in both sets; the numbers of shapes vary in both sets; the shapes are white and black in both sets.

Stage 2: both sets contain no rotations, mirror images or direction changes; however, both sets contain a logical repeat: in Set A all the boxes contain four shapes that create three overlaps and the bottom left-hand corner is always blank and in Set B all the boxes contain three shapes that create two overlaps and the top right-hand corner is always blank.

Stage 3: therefore, the solution must be the *Stage 2* characteristic of each box containing four shapes that create three overlaps with the bottom left-hand corner always blank in Set A, and each box containing three shapes that create two overlaps with the top right-hand corner always blank in Set B. Any test shape not meeting the criteria belongs to Neither Set.

Distracters: shapes, numbers of shapes, sizes of shapes and black shading.

Irrelevant: different shapes in both sets.

Answer to question 36 is Set B: the test shape belongs to Set B as there are three shapes that create two overlaps and the top right-hand corner is blank.

Answer to question 37 is Neither Set: the test shape belongs to Neither Set as there are five shapes that create four overlaps which is not a requirement for either set.

Answer to question 38 is Set B: the test shape belongs to Set B as there are three shapes that create two overlaps and the top right-hand corner is blank.

Answer to question 39 is Set A: the test shape belongs to Set A as there are four shapes that create three overlaps and the bottom left-hand corner is blank.

Answer to question 40 is Neither Set: the test shape belongs to Neither Set as it does not contain any overlapping shapes and there are no blank corners.

Questions 41 to 45

Rationale

Stage 1: the shapes in Set A include a cross, crescent, octagon, triangle, circle and oval, and hearts, rectangles, stars and squares; the shapes in Set B include a hexagon, rectangle and a diamond, and stars, crescents, circles, squares, hearts and ovals; the sizes of the shapes differ in both sets; the numbers of shapes vary in both sets; the shapes are black and white in both sets.

Stage 2: both sets contain no rotations, mirror images or direction changes; however, both sets contain a logical repeat: in Set A all the boxes contain at least one black and one white heart and in Set B all the boxes contain at least two black stars and one white star.

Stage 3: therefore, the solution must be the *Stage 2* characteristic of each box containing at least one black and one white heart in Set A, and each box containing at least two black stars and one white star in Set B. Note, the emphasis is on 'at least' – any test shape containing more than the required number of hearts or stars still meets the criteria for that set. Any test shape not meeting the criteria belongs to Neither Set.

Distracters: shapes, numbers of shapes, sizes of shapes and positions of shapes.

Irrelevant: overlapping or touching shapes and the use of the same shape in some boxes.

Answer to question 41 is Neither Set: the test shape belongs to Neither Set as the shape includes at least one black and one white heart *and* at least two black stars and one white star, so it has the characteristics of both sets (and therefore belongs exclusively to neither).

Answer to question 42 is Set B: the test shape belongs to Set B as there are at least two black stars and one white star.

Answer to question 43 is Neither Set: the test shape belongs to Neither Set as it does not meet the minimum requirement of appropriately coloured hearts or stars for either set.

Answer to question 44 is Set B: the test shape belongs to Set B as there are at least two black stars and one white star.

Answer to question 45 is Set A: the test shape belongs to Set A as there is at least one black and one white heart.

Questions 46 to 50

Rationale
Stage 1: the shapes in Set A contain four playing cards, of which two are spades and two are clubs; Set B also contains four playing cards, of which two are spades and two are clubs. As no picture playing cards are used, the 'ace' is always low, i.e. value of 'one'.

Stage 2: in Set A the two clubs are diagonally opposite from top left to bottom right and the two spades are diagonally opposite from top right to bottom left; the cards are all odd numbers and total to an even number; the highest value card in each row of the box is always a spade and always top right and bottom left: in Set B the two clubs are diagonally opposite from top right to bottom left and the two spades are diagonally opposite from top left to bottom right; the spades are all odd numbers and the clubs are all even numbers, and total to an even number; the highest value card in each row of the box is always a spade and always top left and bottom right.

Stage 3: therefore, the solution must be the *Stage 2* characteristic as detailed above for each set. Any test shape not meeting the criteria belongs to Neither Set.

Distracters: repeats of the same card in any one box.

Irrelevant: repeats of the same cards in both sets.

Answer to question 46 is Set A: the test shape belongs to Set A as the two clubs are diagonally opposite from top left to bottom right and the two spades are diagonally opposite from top right to bottom left; the cards are all odd numbers and total to an even number; the highest value card in each row of the square is always a spade and always top right and bottom left.

Answer to question 47 is Set B: the test shape belongs to Set B as the two clubs are diagonally opposite from top right to bottom left and the two spades are diagonally opposite from top left to bottom right; the spades are all odd numbers and the clubs are all even numbers, and total to an even number; the highest value card in each row of the box is a spade.

Answer to question 48 is Neither Set: the test shape belongs to Neither Set as it contains three club cards and, therefore, can be eliminated immediately.

Answer to question 49 is Neither Set: the test shape belongs to Neither Set as the cards total to an odd number which is the only part of the criteria missing in order to belong to Set A.

Answer to question 50 is Set A: the test shape belongs to Set A as the two clubs are diagonally opposite from top left to bottom right and the two spades are diagonally opposite from top right to bottom left; the cards are all odd numbers and total to an even number; the highest value card in each row of the box is a spade. The repeat of the five of spades is a distracter.

Questions 51 to 55

Rationale

Stage 1: the shapes and symbols in Set A include a rhomboid and triangles, squares, pentagons, arrows and stars; Set B includes a star, cross, rhomboid, diamond and a hexagon and squares, pentagons, triangles, octagons and arrows; the sizes of the shapes vary in both sets; the numbers of shapes vary in both sets; the shapes are grey and white in Set A and shaded and white in Set B.

Stage 2: both sets contain no rotations, mirror images or direction changes; however, both sets contain a logical repeat: in all the boxes in Set A, double the total number of sides of the white shapes added to the total number of sides of the grey shapes equals 26 sides; in all the boxes in Set B, double the total number of sides of the shaded shapes added to the total number of sides of the white shapes equals 30 sides.

Stage 3: therefore, the solution must be the *Stage 2* characteristic of the total number of sides, where grey shapes are counted singly and white shapes are doubled in Set A and where shaded shapes are doubled and white shapes are counted singly in Set B. Any test shape not meeting the criteria belongs to Neither Set.

Distracters: shapes, sizes of shapes and the numbers of shapes.

Irrelevant: different shapes in both sets.

Answer to question 51 is Neither Set: the test shape belongs to Neither Set as the only possibility could be Set B and looking at the criteria for Set B the total number of sides adds to 25, not 30.

Answer to question 52 is Neither Set: the test shape belongs to Neither Set as the only possibility could be Set A and looking at the criteria for Set A the total number of sides adds to 36, not 26.

Answer to question 53 is Set B: the test shape belongs to Set B as the sides of the shaded hexagon (6) doubled equals 12, added to the 8 sides of the white star, the 5 sides of the arrow and the 5 sides of the pentagon totals 30.

Answer to question 54 is Set A: the test shape belongs to Set A as the sides of the white rhomboid (4) and arrow (5) doubled equals 18, added to the 5 sides of the grey arrow and the 3 sides of the triangle totals 26.

Answer to question 55 is Set A: the test shape belongs to Set A as the sides of the white pentagon (5) and the hexagon (6) doubled equals 22, added to the 4 sides of the grey diamond totals 26.

Questions 56 to 60

Rationale

Stage 1: the shapes and symbols in Set A include a star, plaque and a triangle and hearts, crosses, squares, circles and arrows; Set B includes a triangle, heart, plaque, arrow, hexagon, cross and a pentagon and stars, circles, squares, rectangles and ovals; the sizes of the shapes vary in both sets; the numbers of shapes vary in both sets; the shapes are white in both sets, but there are more shapes in Set A.

Stage 2: both sets contain no rotations, mirror images or direction changes; however, both sets contain a logical repeat: in Set A all the boxes contain at least one shape which contains two more shapes within each other and in Set B all the boxes contain at least one shape which has one more shape within it; this is still a logical repeat even when the boxes contain more than one cluster of shapes.

Stage 3: therefore, the solution must be the *Stage 2* characteristic of one shape which contains two more shapes within each other in Set A and one shape which has one more shape within it in Set B. Any test shape not meeting the criteria belongs to Neither Set.

Distracters: shapes and the number of groupings of shapes.

Irrelevant: different shapes in both sets.

Answer to question 56 is Set A: the test shape belongs to Set A as it contains a shape which contains two more shapes within each other.

Answer to question 57 is Set B: the test shape belongs to Set B as it contains a shape which has one more shape within it.

Answer to question 58 is Neither Set: the test shape belongs to Neither Set as one of the shapes does not contain another shape.

Answer to question 59 is Neither Set: the test shape belongs to Neither Set as one shape contains one other shape and the second shape contains two more shapes – this test shape has the characteristics of both sets (and therefore belongs exclusively to neither).

Answer to question 60 is Set A: the test shape belongs to Set A as it contains a shape which contains two more shapes within each other.

Questions 61 to 65

Rationale

Stage 1: the shapes and symbols in Set A include an octagon, crescent, cross, hexagon, star, heart, diamond and a pentagon and circles, rectangles, triangles and arrows; Set B includes a circle, pentagon, trapezium, irregular shape and a square and stars, rectangles, triangles and arrows; the sizes of the shapes vary in both sets; the numbers of shapes vary in both sets; the shapes are white, grey and black in both sets.

Stage 2: both sets contain no rotations, mirror images or direction changes; however, both sets contain a logical repeat: in Set A all the boxes contain several circles, the number of which equals half the number of sides of any straight-sided shapes and in Set B all the boxes contain several stars, the number of which is equal to the number of right angles within any of the other shapes.

Stage 3: therefore, the solution must be the *Stage 2* characteristic of a number of circles which equals half the number of sides of any straight-sided shapes in Set A and a number of stars which is equal to the number of right angles within any of the other shapes in Set B. Any test shape not meeting the criteria belongs to Neither Set.

Distracters: grey and black shading and shapes within other shapes.

Irrelevant: curved shapes other than circles in Set A and curved shapes in Set B.

Answer to question 61 is Set B: the test shape belongs to Set B as there are 8 stars and 8 right angles.

Answer to question 62 is Neither Set: the test shape belongs to Neither Set as there are 20 sides to the straight shapes and only 5 circles instead of 10, therefore it cannot belong to Set A; in addition the requirement for Set B of 4 stars to match the 4 right angles is not met.

Answer to question 63 is Set A: the test shape belongs to Set A as there are 10 circles to the 20 sides of the straight-sided shapes; note the crescent is irrelevant.

Answer to question 64 is Set B: the test shape belongs to Set B as there are 5 stars which equals the 5 right angles; note the crescents and heart are irrelevant.

Answer to question 65 is Set A: the test shape belongs to Set A as there are 6 circles to the 12 sides of the straight-sided shapes.

Chapter 11
The Decision Analysis subtest

This chapter will help you to:

- understand the purpose and the format of the Decision Analysis subtest;
- prepare for the Decision Analysis subtest using general decision analysis questions;
- test your knowledge and understanding of decision analysis-type questions;
- identify those decision analysis skills where development is required.

Introduction

Pearson VUE describes the purpose of this subtest as follows.

The Decision Analysis subtest assesses candidates' ability to decipher and make sense of coded information. You will be presented with a scenario and a significant amount of information together with items that become progressively more complex and ambiguous. The judgements that are required cannot be based on logical deduction alone and this simulates the realities of real-world decision-making where decisions cannot always be made with all the information neatly accessible in one place.

What are decision analysis tests?

Decision analysis tests are, as their name suggests, a measure of an individual's quality of decision-making, both in respect of the adequacy of the decision and the promptness with which the decision has been taken. The behavioural indicators implicit within decision analysis include the ability to identify the relevant information, analyse the facts and consider all the issues, promptness in making the decisions and basing decisions on a reasoned consideration of the evidence.

Decision analysis often forms part of a number of dimensions being assessed in the recruitment process and in other types of selection and, in particular, for situations requiring managerial skills. The dimensions can be assessed either through a series of exercises and scenarios or by the use of psychometric tests. However, the use of such tests specifically to determine an individual's ability to make decisions is unusual.

Decision Analysis subtest

Before attempting the practice questions based on the approach taken in the UKCAT, you should find it beneficial to work through the following questions. The scenario and items have been formatted along the lines to be used in the UKCAT, and the answers and the rationales for the correct answers follow each question.

Scenario, response formats and example questions

The scenario for a decision analysis test can contain information in a variety of formats. However, in view of the time constraints imposed for this subtest, it is probable that the information contained in the scenario will be reasonably short and specific, and is likely to include an initial paragraph of explanatory text, a list of codes in tabular or similar format and a couple of worked examples. New information will be added at some stage during the test to add to the complexity of the items. This will be in the form of additional codes with a brief explanation. The information and examples will be accessible throughout the test.

The scenario provided by the Pearson VUE website, in their practice test, has an explanatory paragraph followed by information in a tabular format to which new information is added for the final example. The practice test information consists of a series of codes from which the items have been taken. Essentially, this requires the respondent to identify the words contained within part of the code and to see which answer options best fit those particular words.

The explanatory paragraph directs the respondent to make 'your best judgement' in selecting the correct option or options. 'Best judgement' means your judgement based solely on the codes themselves and not on what you might consider to be reasonable. This is not dissimilar to the Verbal Reasoning subtest in that you need to focus on the information provided and not use your knowledge or experience in answering any of the items.

Codes may be combined to produce a new but related concept (for example, the codes of 'air' and 'ice' could combine to become 'snow'). In addition, you will be asked to make more subtle judgements, particularly when the ordering of the codes is not obvious or when some codes appear to be missing.

In line with the Pearson VUE format for the Decision Analysis subtest, the scenarios used both in the example below and in the following practice test are in the style of coded information. Where appropriate, the requirement of selecting more than one option is clearly identified.

Example questions

The following examples are intended to go from the simple to the complex, commencing with a simple code and building into codes with both specific and additional information, increasing the level of complexity.

Example scenario 1

A group of explorers in the Amazon rain forest stumble upon what appears to be the ruined site of an ancient civilisation. In exploring one of the ruined buildings, they find a tablet of stone with what appears to be a coded message. What does it mean?

100504E   5OO5ES   65050A

This coded message can be answered by changing the numbers to roman numerals to reveal the meaning:

CLIVE LOVES VILLA

This example is used to introduce you to the world of cryptography (codes and ciphers) where use is often made of cryptograms (i.e. coded messages). However, you will be pleased to hear that the UKCAT does not require you to break a code or cipher. The scenario will provide you with both the code and its meaning. Although this sounds simple, it is not necessarily so – particularly when you are under time pressure to make prompt decisions. We'll therefore look at a scenario and items similar to those used in the UKCAT.

Example scenario 2

Counter-intelligence codes

In the secret world of counter-intelligence it is not unusual for messages between agencies and agents to be encrypted. In the modern era this encryption can be extremely sophisticated but, for the purposes of this scenario, a method of letter, number and symbol substitution is used. The codes used by one counter-intelligence agency within Europe are presented in the table below. The information from the codes may not always be complete, but you are asked to make your best judgement based on this information and not on what you might consider to be reasonable.

Table: counter-intelligence codes

Operating codes	Routine codes
α = delay	01 = explosive
β = previous	02 = today
γ = cancel	03 = sun
δ = negative	04 = rain
ε = increase	05 = agent
ζ = hot	06 = public
η = opposite	07 = smoke
υ = include	08 = safe
	09 = building
	10 = drop
	11 = tonight
	12 = dark
	13 = weapon
	14 = abort
	15 = secret
	16 = operation

Opposite are two examples of how the codes work.

Example item 1

Examine the following coded message:

α, 16, 03, 04

The code combines the words 'delay', 'operation', 'sun', 'rain'.

Now examine the following sentences and try to determine which is the most likely interpretation of the code:

A   The operation is delayed due to sun and rain.

B   The operation is delayed due to sun.

C   The operation is delayed due to rain.

D   Delay the operation until it is dry.

E   Delay operation rainbow.

All the options contain elements of the codes. However, a decision has to be made as to which of the options provides the most likely interpretation.

Answer and rationale

Option E 'Delay operation rainbow' is the correct answer as it uses all the codes. Note 'sun' and 'rain' combine to make 'rainbow'.

Option A uses all the codes but it is not likely that the operation would be delayed for 'sun' and 'rain'. Look for a better option.

Option B does not use the code 'rain'.

Option C does not use the code 'sun'.

Option D introduces the word 'dry', which could relate to 'sun', but it does not use the code 'rain'.

Example item 2

Examine the following coded message.

06, 09, ε(08η), 11

The code combines the words 'public', 'building', 'increase (safe opposite)', 'tonight'.

Now examine the following sentences and try to determine which is the most likely interpretation of the code.

A The public building is safe tonight.

B The public building is dangerous.

C People in the cinema are very safe tonight.

D People in the building are in extreme danger today.

E People in the cinema are in extreme danger tonight.

All the options contain elements of the codes. However, a decision has to be made as to which of the options provides the most likely interpretation.

Answer and rationale

Option E 'People in the cinema are in extreme danger tonight' is the correct answer as it uses all the codes. 'Public' can be 'people', a 'cinema' is a 'building', 'extreme danger' is an 'increase of the opposite of safe'.

Option A does not 'increase the opposite of safe'.

Option B does not use the word 'tonight' and it does not increase 'danger'.

Option C increases 'safe' rather than the 'opposite of safe'.

Option D introduces the code 'today', which is not used.

The following two examples will include new information, as detailed below.

New information added – codes for specialisms and personality traits

The Head of Counter-intelligence has appointed new agents and they use a more sophisticated coding system that will impact on the previous codes.

Table: counter-intelligence codes including codes for specialisms and personality

Operating codes	Routine codes	Specialist codes	Personality codes
α = delay	01 = explosive	A = full	101 = emotional
β = previous	02 = today	B = wound	102 = assertive
γ = cancel	03 = sun	C = mortal	103 = trusting
δ = negative	04 = rain	D = fast	104 = confident
ε = increase	05 = agent	E = enjoyable	105 = practical
ζ = hot	06 = public		106 = volatile
η = opposite	07 = smoke		
υ = include	08 = safe		
	09 = building		
	10 = drop		
	11 = tonight		
	12 = dark		
	13 = weapon		
	14 = abort		
	15 = secret		
	16 = operation		

The following example has the codes in a different order from the solution.

Example item 3

Examine the following coded message.

101η, 101, 05, 102, 06, 106

The code combines the words 'emotional opposite', 'emotional', 'agent', 'assertive', 'public', 'volatile'.

Now examine the following sentences and try to determine which is the most likely interpretation of the code.

A   Agents are assertive and volatile with the public.

B   The public are calm in volatile situations.

C   People react in an emotionally volatile way with assertive agents.

D   Agents need to be assertive and emotional when dealing with calm people.

E   Agents need to be assertive and calm when dealing with emotionally volatile people.

All the options contain elements of the codes. However, a decision has to be made as to which of the options provides the most likely interpretation.

Answer and rationale

Option E 'Agents need to be assertive and calm when dealing with emotionally volatile people' is the correct answer as it uses all the codes. 'Public' can be 'people', 'calm' is the 'opposite of emotional'.

Option A does not use 'emotional opposite' (calm) or 'emotional'.

Option B does not use the words 'agent' and 'assertive'.

Option C does not use 'emotional opposite' (calm).

Option D is possible as it uses all the codes, but it is not the most likely solution. Look for a better option.

The following example has two options that could be correct and also has some information missing. When you sit the UKCAT you may not be aware that information is missing, but an analysis of the options should make this obvious. You are required to make a logical decision as to what the missing information is.

Example item 4

Examine the following coded message.

Dε, 16, 15, 05, 08, 11

The code combines the words 'fast increase', 'operation', 'secret', 'agent', 'safe', 'tonight'.

Now examine the following sentences and try to determine which is the most likely interpretation of the code.

A   A fast operation will ensure the safety of the public.

B   The secret agent will operate faster.

C   The secret agent is safe tonight following the operation.

D   The agent will have to carry out tonight's secret mission very quickly to ensure the safety of the public.

E   The agent will have to carry out tonight's secret operation very fast to ensure the building is safe.

All the options contain elements of the codes. However, a decision has to be made as to which of the options provides the most likely interpretation.

Answer and rationale

Options D and E could both be correct. Option D 'The agent will have to carry out tonight's secret mission very quickly to ensure the safety of the public' uses all the codes with the addition of the missing information 'public'. The word 'operation' can be 'mission' and 'very fast' can be 'very quickly'. Option E 'The agent will have to carry out tonight's secret operation very fast to ensure the building is safe' uses all the codes with the addition of the missing information 'building'.

Option A includes the addition of the missing information 'public' but it does not increase 'fast' and it does not use the words 'agent' and 'tonight'.

Option B cannot be discounted because it does not add in any missing information, but it can be discounted because it does not use the words 'safe' and 'tonight'.

Option C cannot be discounted because it does not add in any missing information, but it can be discounted because it does not use the word 'fast'.

Decision Analysis practice subtest

The Decision Analysis subtest is an on-screen test that consists of one scenario and 26 associated items. The scenario may contain text, tables and other types of information. The 26 items have five response options and for some items more than one of the options may be correct. Where more than one of the response options is correct this is clearly identified within the item. A period of thirty minutes is allowed for the test, with one minute for instruction and the remaining twenty-nine minutes for items.

If you want to simulate 'test conditions', you are advised to use rough paper to mark down your choice for each of the questions (i.e. A, B, C, D or E). For questions with more than one answer option you will need to note all the appropriate options.

The correct answer and rationale for each of the questions are produced in the section following the practice subtest.

Decision Analysis practice subtest: questions

Intergalactic Space Agency codes

The Intergalactic Space Agency (ISA) is a highly expert team of code breakers. Their main remit is the interception of alien communications in the interests of universal security within the known universe. In order to meet their undertakings, they are required to identify and decipher all intergalactic communications. The ISA is recruiting new agents and has set the following codes as its application test. To pass this test you will be required to interpret the coded questions and select the best option or options from those listed. The information from the codes may not always be complete, but you are asked to make your 'best judgement' based on this information and not on what you might consider to be reasonable.

Table: Intergalactic Space Agency codes

Operating codes	Basic codes
T = opposite	⚹ = me
U = negative	☆ = others
V = unite	◆ = oxygen
W = hot	♣ = hydrogen
X = enlarge	♥ = fire
Y = slow	▲ = Mars
Z = similar	◗ = Moon
	✳ = Sun
	✛ = tonight
	▢ = home
	◉ = see
	→ = ship
	■ = heavy
	? = hard
	✔ = prefer

Below are two examples of how the codes work.

Example item 1

Examine the following coded message.

✴, XW, ⚊, ?, 👁

The code combines the words 'Sun', 'enlarge hot', 'me', 'hard', 'see'.

Now examine the following sentences and try to determine which is the most likely interpretation of the code.

A The Sun is very large and is blinding me.

B The very hot Sun is burning me.

C I like to see hot sunny weather.

D The hot Sun makes me squint.

E The Sun is very hot and I find it hard to see.

All the options contain elements of the codes. However, a decision has to be made as to which of the options provides the most likely interpretation.

Answer and rationale

Option E 'The Sun is very hot and I find it hard to see' is the correct answer as it uses all the codes. Note 'me' can be 'I' and 'enlarge hot' is 'very hot'.

Option A uses 'hard' and 'see', which could combine to make 'blinding', but this option enlarges 'Sun' and does not use the word 'hot'.

Option B introduces the word 'burning' and, although there is a code for 'fire', this is not included. In addition the code 'see' is missing.

Option C uses 'like' and 'weather', which are not code words. 'Sun' could become 'weather' but the code is not used twice.

Option D is almost possible, but 'hot' is not enlarged.

Example item 2

Examine the following coded message.

Ϯ, X(U✔), ❤

The code combines the words 'me', 'enlarge (negative prefer)', 'fire'.

Now examine the following sentences and try to determine which is the most likely interpretation of the code.

A I really like a fire.

B I dislike sitting by the fire at home.

C I am really fiery.

D A big fire suits me.

E I really dislike fire.

All the options contain elements of the codes. However, a decision has to be made as to which of the options provides the most likely interpretation.

Answer and rationale

Option E 'I really dislike fire' is the correct answer as it uses all the codes. 'Me' becomes 'I' and 'enlarge (negative prefer)' becomes 'really dislike'.

Option A uses 'enlarge prefer' instead of 'enlarge (negative prefer)' (dislike).

Option B introduces 'sitting', which is not a code, and 'home', which is not included.

Option C increases 'fire' and does not use 'negative prefer' (dislike).

Option D introduces the word 'big', which could be 'enlarge', but 'suits' is not the opposite of 'prefer'.

New information added – codes for technical aspects and personality traits

The ISA team has identified new codes that will impact on the previous codes.

Table: Intergalactic Space Agency codes including codes for technical aspects and personality traits

Operating codes	Basic codes	Technical codes	Characteristic codes
T = opposite	⚓ = me	501 = warp	901 = warm
U = negative	☆ = others	502 = damage	902 = sociable
V = unite	◆ = oxygen	503 = capacity	903 = aggression
W = hot	♣ = hydrogen	504 = vacuum	904 = tense
X = enlarge	❤ = fire	505 = boost	905 = cynical
Y = slow	▲ = Mars	506 = aliens	
Z = similar	◖ = Moon		
	☀ = Sun		
	✚ = tonight		
	❑ = home		
	👁 = see		
	→ = ship		
	■ = heavy		
	? = hard		
	✔ = prefer		

Question 1

What is the best interpretation of the following coded message?

V(⚓☆), TY, ▲ ◖ ☀ →, ❑, ✚

A   We are going home by spacecraft.

B   Fly me to the Moon tonight.

C   We need a fast spacecraft to get home tonight.

D   A fast spacecraft will get us home.

E   Tonight the spaceship is going to Mars.

Question 2

What is the best interpretation of the following coded message?

♣, ◆, ◆ ♣, ■T

A   Hydrogen and oxygen are heavy gases.

B   Oxygen is lighter than hydrogen.

C   Oxygen and hydrogen are floating gases.

D   Hydrogen and oxygen are light gases.

E   Hydrogen is lighter than oxygen.

Question 3

What would be the best way to encode the following message?

The atmosphere on the Moon makes me light and slow.

A   ◆♣, ◖, ⚘, ■T, Y

B   ◆♣, ◖, ⚘V☆, ■T, Y

C   ◆♣, ◖, ☆, ■T, Y

D   ◆♣, ◖, ⚘, ■, Y

E   ◆♣, ◖, ⚘, ■T, YT

Question 4

What is the best interpretation of the following coded message?

▢, ✳X, XT◉, ◆♣

A   The sunshine at home is blinding.

B   The atmosphere on Earth is good when the Sun shines.

C   Oxygen and hydrogen levels are the opposite on the Sun and Earth.

D   The atmosphere totally obscured the sunshine on Earth.

E   Sunshine is greater at home when the atmosphere is clear.

Question 5

What is the best interpretation of the following coded message?

TW, W, ⚘V☆▢, 901, ◖, ▲

A   Earth is warm, the Moon is cold and Mars is hot.

B   Our home is cold and the Moon and Mars are hot.

C   Earth and the Moon are cold and Mars is hot.

D   Our planet is warm and Mars is hot.

E   Earth and Mars are hot and the Moon is cold.

Question 6

What is the best interpretation of the following coded message?

▢, 𝕏, T▢, 901T, U904, ✔

A   I am anxious when not at home.

B   Home is where I chill out.

C   I like to relax and chill out at home.

D   I prefer to be in a warm home.

E   A warm home is where I like to be.

Question 7

What is the best interpretation of the following coded message?

U♥, 504, 501, →

A   The ship's engines fail to fire in a vacuum.

B   The ship's warp drive is in a vacuum.

C   Firing the ship's engines creates a vacuum.

D   A vacuum is required to fire the ship's engines.

E   The ship's engines only fire in a vacuum.

Question 8

What is the best interpretation of the following coded message?

903, 𝕏☆, 502, 902, V☆

(NB: **Two** options are correct.)

A   Aggressive people do not join social groups.

B   Social groups are marred by aggressive people.

C   Aggression breaks up social groups.

D   Social groups can contain aggressive people.

E   Aggressive people damage social groups.

Question 9

What is the best interpretation of the following coded message?

(901, 902, 903, 904, 905), 506, 506T, UT

A   Humans have positive personalities but aliens are negative.

B   Humans and aliens both have negative personalities.

C   Aliens are warm and sociable, while humans are cynical.

D   Humans and aliens both have positive personalities.

E   Aliens have opposite personalities to humans.

Question 10

What is the best interpretation of the following coded message?

905X, 506T, ◉X, WT,   ▲506

A   Martians are cold and cynical.

B   Earthlings are cold and cynical compared to Martians.

C   Martians are viewed with cold cynicism by earthlings.

D   Martians are seen as cynical.

E   Earthlings and Martians are cold and cynical.

Question 11

What is the best interpretation of the following coded message?

501, Z→, 505X, XX

A   The ship's warp has been increased.

B   The craft is boosted by the warp drive.

C   Increased power is what the ship needs.

D Extra warp would increase the ship's speed.

E The craft's drive and boosters have been increased.

Question 12

What is the best interpretation of the following coded message?

🧍☆, →, X502, ◆♣, ✳(T■)

A Oxygen, hydrogen and sunlight damage our spaceship.

B Hydrogen is lighter than oxygen on our Sun.

C Our ship to the Sun runs on oxygen and hydrogen.

D The sunlight and elements destroy our spaceship.

E Oxygen and hydrogen are destructive elements.

Question 13

What is the best interpretation of the following coded message?

✓, 🧍☆, ◆, T◆, U✓, T506

A Humans prefer oxygen.

B Humans do not like carbon dioxide, as they prefer oxygen.

C Aliens prefer carbon dioxide to oxygen.

D Humans like carbon dioxide and oxygen.

E Aliens do not like oxygen, as they prefer carbon dioxide.

Question 14

What is the best interpretation of the following coded message?
506, 902, 503, 🧍

A I am sociable with aliens.

B I have the capacity to be aggressive in dealing with aliens.

C I have the ability to be sociable and aggressive in dealing with aliens.

D Aliens do not have the capacity to be sociable and aggressive with me.

E I have the same capacity of character as aliens.

Question 15

What is the best interpretation of the following coded message?
☆, 506, T903
(NB: **Two** options are correct.)

A Other people make aliens aggressive.

B Aliens are peace-loving people.

C Aliens are gentle unlike other people.

D Aliens are a non-aggressive race.

E Others are aggressive to aliens.

Question 16

What is the best interpretation of the following coded message?
 ?TU, VT, 506, 506T
(NB: **Two** options are correct.)

A It's not very easy to separate aliens from non-aliens.

B Aliens are hard and should be kept separate.

C It's quite hard to separate aliens from non-aliens.

D It's easy to unite aliens and non-aliens.

E Aliens and non-aliens cannot be separated.

Question 17

What is the best interpretation of the following coded message?
V, 905T, →, ☆U

A Trust the others with the ship.

B The others are cynical about uniting with the ship.

C The others on the ship cannot be trusted.

D Trust nobody with the ship.

E The others will not be joining the ship.

Question 18

What is the best interpretation of the following coded message?
◆U, ▲, ◖, ✳, Z, XZT, WTW

(NB: **Two** options are correct.)

A   Oxygen levels and temperatures on Mars, the Sun and the Moon are similar.

B   Oxygen levels are similarly low on Mars, the Sun and the Moon but the temperatures vary greatly.

C   The lack of oxygen on Mars, the Sun and the Moon makes the temperatures vary.

D   Mars, the Sun and the Moon are very hot and devoid of oxygen.

E   The lack of oxygen on Mars, the Sun and the Moon is similar but the temperatures are very different.

Question 19

What is the best interpretation of the following coded message?
506T, 901, 902, 903, 904, 905, U, UT, YTY, ▲X

A   The moods of humans are influenced by Mars.

B   Negative and positive characteristics can be found in humans and aliens alike.

C   The movement of the planets has a positive or negative impact on human characteristics.

D   Human characteristics are opposite to aliens from Mars.

E   Fast moving planets influence human personality traits.

Question 20

Which **two** of the following would be the most useful additions to the codes when attempting to convey the following message?

The cold, thin air on Jupiter makes me very sleepy.

A   planet

B   tired

C   chilly

D   narrow

E   atmosphere

Question 21

What is the best interpretation of the following coded message?

X V(903, 904), 🚶, 506, V(🚶☆), 502, □

A We get very tense when aliens attack our planet.

B I get very angry when people break into my house.

C It makes me very hostile when aliens attack our planet.

D The planet is being damaged by hostile aliens.

E Aliens are aggressive and damage my house.

Question 22

What would be the best way to encode the following message?

The fire damage to the warp drive is a very tense situation for us.

A ❤, 502, 904X, 506, 🚶V☆

B 🚶V☆, ❤, 502, 904X, 506

C 🚶V☆, ❤, 502, 904, 501

D ❤, 502, 904X, 501, 🚶☆

E 🚶V☆, ❤, 502, 904X, 501

Question 23

What is the best interpretation of the following coded message?

➜, X❤, XT902, 506, V(🚶☆)

A The aliens were very unfriendly and fired at our ship.

B The fire on our ship was started by aliens.

C We fired at the unfriendly alien ship.

D The alien ship was subjected to unfriendly fire.

E Firing at our ship was not very sociable.

Question 24

What would be the best way to encode the following message?

Martians have the capacity to be both friendly and aggressive just like us.

A   503, ▲506, 902, 903, V(🏃☆), Z

B   ▲, 506, 503, V(902 903), ☆, Z

C   ▲506, V(902 903), V(🏃☆), Z

D   503, ▲506, V(902 903), V(🏃☆), Z

E   ✔, ▲506, V(902 903), V(🏃☆), Z

Question 25

What is the best interpretation of the following coded message?
V(Z♣ ❤), ☆, →, ■X, 501

A   Hydrogen is heavier than oxygen and warps the ship.

B   Some gases are heavier than others and affect the ship's speed.

C   The warp speed of the ship is affected by gases.

D   Gases like oxygen and hydrogen affect the ship's speed.

E   The ship's warp drive runs on gas.

Question 26

Which **two** of the following would be the most useful additions to the codes when attempting to convey the following message?

The red and orange glow from Mars reflects off our ship.

A   mirror

B   ember

C   bounces

D   shine

E   colours

Decision Analysis practice subtest: answers

Question number	Correct response
1	Option C
2	Option D
3	Option A
4	Option D
5	Option A
6	Option C
7	Option A
8	Option B & E
9	Option D
10	Option C
11	Option E
12	Option D
13	Option B
14	Option C
15	Options B & D
16	Options A & C
17	Option D
18	Options B & E
19	Option C
20	Options B & D
21	Option C
22	Option E
23	Option A
24	Option D
25	Option B
26	Options C & E

Decision Analysis practice subtest: explanation of answers

Question 1

Answer and rationale
V(⟨ ⟩), TY, ▲◖✳→, ▢, ✚

The code combines the words 'unite me others', 'opposite slow', 'Mars Moon Sun ship', 'home', 'tonight'.

Option C 'We need a fast spacecraft to get home tonight' is the correct answer as it uses all the codes with, 'unite me others' being used as 'we', 'opposite slow' being used as 'fast', 'Mars Moon Sun ship' being used as 'spacecraft'.

Option A has failed to use the code 'opposite slow' as 'fast' and has omitted the code 'tonight'.

Option B has not used the code 'unite me others' as 'we', or the code 'home' and 'Mars Moon Sun ship' has been poorly interpreted as 'fly me to the Moon'.

Option D has interpreted 'unite me others' as 'us' which is plausible; however, the code 'tonight' has not been used.

Option E has used the code 'Mars' twice and has failed to use the code 'home'.

Question 2

Answer and rationale
♣, ♦, ♦♣, ■T

The code combines the words 'hydrogen', 'oxygen', 'oxygen hydrogen', 'heavy opposite'.

Option D 'Hydrogen and oxygen are light gases' is the correct answer as it uses all the codes with, 'oxygen hydrogen' being used as 'gases' and 'heavy opposite' being used as 'light'.

Option A has failed to use 'opposite' with 'heavy'.

Option B has enlarged 'heavy opposite' to 'lighter' and has not used the code 'oxygen hydrogen'.

Option C has used the code 'heavy opposite' as 'floating', which is a poor interpretation.

Option E has enlarged 'heavy opposite' to 'lighter' and has not used the code 'oxygen hydrogen'.

Question 3

Answer and rationale

Option A would be the best way to encode the message 'The atmosphere on the Moon makes me light and slow': ◆♣, ◖, ⵣ, ▮T, Y

This option has the correct codes by using ◆♣ 'oxygen hydrogen' as 'atmosphere', and ▮T 'heavy opposite' as 'light'.

Option B has used the code for ⵣ V ☆ 'me unite others', instead of the code for 'me'.

Option C has used the code for 'others', instead of the code for 'me'.

Option D has not used the code 'opposite' with the code for 'heavy'.

Option E has used the code YT 'slow opposite', instead of just the code for 'slow'.

Question 4

Answer and rationale

▢, ✳X, XT👁, ◆♣

The code combines the words 'home', 'Sun enlarge', 'enlarge opposite see', 'oxygen hydrogen'.

Option D 'The atmosphere totally obscured the sunshine on Earth' is the correct answer as it uses all the codes with, 'home' being used as 'Earth', 'Sun enlarge' being used as 'sunshine', 'enlarge opposite see' being used as 'totally obscured' and 'oxygen hydrogen' being used as 'atmosphere'.

Option A has not used the code 'oxygen hydrogen' – otherwise it would have been a plausible interpretation with 'enlarge opposite see' being used as 'blinding'.

Option B has not used the code 'enlarge opposite see' and has added the word 'good'.

Option C has applied the code 'opposite' to levels of oxygen and hydrogen instead of to the code 'see'.

Option E has not used the code 'opposite' with 'see' and has therefore misinterpreted the code as 'clear'.

Question 5

Answer and rationale

TW, W, ⵣ V☆▢, 901, ◖, ▲

The code combines the words 'opposite hot', 'hot', 'me unite others home', 'warm', 'Moon', 'Mars'.

Option A 'Earth is warm, the Moon is cold and Mars is hot' is the correct answer as it uses all the codes with, 'opposite hot' being used as 'cold' and 'me unite others home' being used as 'our home' which in turn is interpreted as 'Earth'.

Option B has failed to interpret 'our home' as 'Earth' and has omitted the code 'warm'.

Option C has not used the code 'warm'.

Option D has interpreted 'our home' as 'our planet' and has not used the codes 'warm' or 'cold'.

Option E has not used the code 'warm'.

Question 6

Answer and rationale

⬜, 🕴, T⬜, 901T, U904, ✔

The code combines the words 'home', 'me', 'opposite home', 'warm opposite', 'negative tense', 'prefer'.

Option C 'I like to relax and chill out at home' is the correct answer as it uses all the codes with, 'opposite home' being used as 'out', 'warm opposite' being used as 'chill', 'negative tense' being used as 'relax' and 'prefer' being used as 'like'.

Option A has used 'negative tense' as 'anxious', has not used 'home' twice and has not used the codes 'opposite warm' and 'prefer'.

Option B has not used the code 'opposite' with 'warm' and has not used the code 'opposite home'.

Option D has not used the code 'negative tense'.

Option E has not used the code 'opposite home'.

Question 7

Answer and rationale

U❤, 504, 501, →

The code combines the words 'negative fire', 'vacuum', 'warp', 'ship'.

Option A 'The ship's engines fail to fire in a vacuum' is the correct answer as it uses all the codes with, 'negative fire' being used as 'fail to fire', 'warp' being used as 'engines'.

Option B has failed to use the code 'negative fire'.

Option C has used the code 'negative fire' as 'firing' which is incorrect.

Option D has failed to make the code 'fire' into 'negative fire'.

Option E has also failed to make the code 'fire' into 'negative fire'.

Question 8

Answer and rationale
903, 人☆, 502, 902, V☆

(NB: **Two** options are correct.)

The code combines the words 'aggression', 'me others', 'damage', 'sociable', 'unite others'.

Option B 'Social groups are marred by aggressive people' and Option E 'Aggressive people damage social groups' are the correct answers as both contain all the codes. Both options have used 'aggression' as 'aggressive, 'me others' as 'people', 'sociable' as 'social' and 'unite others' as 'groups'. Option B has used the code 'damage' as 'marred', otherwise both options have the same interpretation.

Option A has failed to use the code 'damage' and has inserted 'do not join'.

Option C has used the code 'damage' as 'breaks up' and has omitted the code 'me others' as 'people'.

Option D has failed to use the code 'damage' and has inserted 'can contain'.

Question 9

Answer and rationale
(901, 902, 903, 904, 905), 506, 506T, UT

The code combines the words 'warm', 'sociable', 'aggression', 'tense', 'cynical', 'aliens', 'aliens opposite', 'negative opposite'.

Option D 'Humans and aliens both have positive personalities' is the correct answer as it uses all the codes with, 'warm', 'sociable', 'aggression', 'tense', 'cynical', being combined as 'personalities', 'aliens opposite' being used as 'humans' and 'negative opposite' being used as 'positive'.

Option A has wrongly assigned positive and negative personalities to humans and aliens respectively, and has added an additional 'negative' code.

Option B has used the code 'negative' instead of 'negative opposite' as 'positive'.

Option C has wrongly assigned some characteristics to aliens and some to humans.

Option E has used the code 'opposite' in isolation and has also assigned opposite personalities to aliens and humans.

Question 10

Answer and rationale

905X, 506T, ⟨👁X, WT, ▲506

The code combines the words 'cynical enlarge', 'aliens opposite', 'see enlarged', 'hot opposite', 'Mars aliens'.

Option C 'Martians are viewed with cold cynicism by earthlings' is the correct answer as it uses all the codes with, 'cynical enlarge' being used as 'cynicism', 'aliens opposite' being used as 'earthlings', 'see enlarge' being used as 'viewed', 'hot opposite' being used as 'cold' and 'Mars aliens' being used as 'Martians'.

Option A has not used the codes 'aliens opposite', 'see enlarge' and has not enlarged 'cynical'.

Option B has not used the code 'see enlarge' and has not enlarged 'cynical'.

Option D has not used the codes 'aliens opposite' and 'hot opposite'.

Option E has not used the code 'see enlarge' and has not enlarged 'cynical'.

Question 11

Answer and rationale

501, Z→, 505X, XX

The code combines the words 'warp', 'similar ship', 'boost enlarge', 'enlarge enlarge'.

Option E 'The craft's drive and boosters have been increased' is the correct answer as it uses all the codes with, 'warp' being used as 'drive', 'similar ship' being used as 'craft's', 'boost enlarge' being used as 'boosters' and 'enlarge enlarge' being used as 'increased'.

Option A has used the code 'ship' instead of 'ship similar' and has not used the code 'boost enlarge'.

Option B has not used the code 'enlarge enlarge' and has used the code 'warp' twice.

Option C has used the code 'ship' instead of 'ship similar' and has combined 'warp' and 'boost enlarge' as 'power'.

Option D has used the code 'enlarge enlarge' separately as 'extra' and 'increase' and has used the code 'boost enlarge' as 'speed'.

Question 12

Answer and rationale
🚶☆, →, X502, ◆♣, ☀(T▪)

The code combines the words 'me others', 'ship', 'enlarge damage', 'oxygen hydrogen', 'Sun opposite heavy'.

Option D 'The sunlight and elements destroy our spaceship' is the correct answer as it uses all the codes with, 'me others' being used as 'our', 'ship' being used as 'spaceship', 'enlarge damage' being used as 'destroy', 'oxygen hydrogen' being used as 'elements' and 'Sun opposite heavy' being used as 'sunlight'.

Option A has not used the code 'enlarge damage' as 'destroy', and is therefore a misinterpretation of this code, otherwise it would be a plausible interpretation.

Option B has not used the code 'ship' or the code 'enlarge damage' and has split 'Sun opposite heavy' as 'lighter' and 'Sun'.

Option C has not used the code 'enlarge damage' and has used the code 'Sun' instead of 'Sun opposite heavy'.

Option E has not used the codes 'me others', 'ship' and 'Sun opposite heavy', and it has used the code 'oxygen hydrogen' as 'elements'.

Question 13

Answer and rationale
✓, 🚶☆, ◆, T◆, U✓, T506

The code combines the words 'prefer', 'me others', 'oxygen', 'opposite oxygen', 'negative prefer', 'opposite aliens'.

Option B 'Humans do not like carbon dioxide, as they prefer oxygen' is the correct answer as it uses all the codes with, 'me others' being used as 'they', 'opposite oxygen' being used as 'carbon dioxide', 'negative prefer' being used as 'do not like' and 'opposite aliens' being used as 'humans'.

Option A has not used the codes 'negative prefer' and 'opposite oxygen'.

Option C has not used the codes 'me others', 'negative prefer' and has used the code 'aliens' instead of 'opposite aliens'.

Option D has not used the code 'me others' and 'negative prefer'.

Option E has not used the code 'opposite aliens' otherwise it could have been a possible interpretation.

Question 14

Answer and rationale

506, 902, 503, ⟨symbol⟩

The code combines the words 'aliens', 'sociable', 'capacity', 'me'.

Option C 'I have the ability to be sociable and aggressive in dealing with aliens' is the correct answer even though it contains the word 'aggressive', which is not shown in the codes. This is an instance where you are being asked to make a more subtle judgement when some code(s) appear to be missing. In this instance it is necessary to consider carefully all the options before determining that this is the correct one.

Option A does not contain the code 'capacity' and can therefore be eliminated.

Option B does not contain the code 'sociable' though it has introduced another code 'aggression'. On the basis of it not containing one of the codes, it can be eliminated.

Option D contains all the codes but again has included another code 'aggression'. In addition, the option states 'do not have' and for this there would need to be some other 'negative' code. Because two new codes would be required as opposed to the one in Option C, this answer can be eliminated.

Option E is incorrect as it mentions 'character', which would include all the 'characteristics', and not just 'sociable' or even 'aggression'.

Question 15

Answer and rationale

⟨star symbol⟩, 506, T903

(NB: **Two** options are correct.)

The code combines the words 'others', 'aliens', 'opposite aggression'.

Option B 'Aliens are peace-loving people' and Option D 'Aliens are a non-aggressive race' are the correct answers. Both options contain all the codes and use appropriate terms for the codes 'opposite aggression' and 'others' – namely, 'peace-loving people' and 'non-aggressive race', respectively.

Option A does not take into account the code 'opposite aggression'.

Option C uses all the codes but adds further information that is not contained in the combinations (i.e. 'unlike other people').

Option E does not take into account the code 'opposite aggression'.

Question 16

Answer and rationale
?TU, VT, 506, 506T

(NB: **Two** options are correct.)

The code combines the words 'hard opposite (negative)', 'unite opposite', 'aliens', 'aliens opposite'.

Option A 'It's not very easy to separate aliens from non-aliens' and Option C 'It's quite hard to separate aliens from non-aliens' are the correct answers as both contain all the codes. Option A and Option C have interpreted 'hard opposite (negative)' as 'not very easy' and 'quite hard' respectively, both of which could be correct.

Option B has not used the 'aliens opposite' code to become 'non-aliens'.

Option D has not used the 'hard opposite (negative)' code to become 'not very easy' or 'quite hard'. Instead it has used this code as 'easy'.

Option E has not used the code 'hard opposite (negative)' code to become 'not very easy' or 'quite hard'. Instead it has introduced the word 'cannot'.

Question 17

Answer and rationale
V, 905T, →, ☆U

The code combines the words 'unite', 'cynical opposite', 'ship', 'others negative'.

Option D 'Trust nobody with the ship' is the correct answer as it uses all the codes. 'Unite' becomes 'with', 'cynical opposite' becomes 'trust' and 'others negative' becomes 'nobody'. Note, the codes do not have to be in the same order as the most logical interpretation.

Option A has not used the 'others negative' code to become 'nobody'. Instead it has used the 'others' code.

Option B has not used the 'others negative' code to become 'nobody'. Instead it has used the 'others' code. In addition, it has not used the 'cynical opposite' to become 'trust'. Instead it has used the 'cynical' code.

Option C has not used the 'others negative' code to become 'nobody'. Instead it has used the 'others' code.

Option E has not used the 'others negative' code to become 'nobody'. Instead it has used the 'others' code. In addition, it has used the 'unite' code as 'joining' instead of 'with'.

Question 18

Answer and rationale

◆U, ▲, ◖, ✳, Z, XZT, WTW

(NB: **Two** options are correct.)

The code combines the words 'oxygen negative', 'Mars', 'Moon', 'Sun', 'similar', '(enlarge) similar opposite', 'hot opposite hot '.

Option B 'Oxygen levels are similarly low on Mars, the Sun and the Moon but the temperatures vary greatly' and Option E 'The lack of oxygen on Mars, the Sun and the Moon is similar but the temperatures are very different' are the correct answers as both contain all the codes. Options B and E have interpreted the 'oxygen negative' code as low levels of oxygen or a lack of oxygen, respectively, both of which could be correct. The code '(enlarge) similar opposite' has been interpreted as 'vary greatly' or 'very different', again both of which could be correct. Both options have used the code 'hot opposite hot' as 'hot and cold' which in turn is interpreted as temperatures.

Option A has not used the code '(enlarge) similar opposite' as 'vary greatly' or 'very different'. Instead it has used the code 'similar'.

Option C has associated the 'oxygen negative' code with the '(enlarge) similar opposite' and the 'hot opposite hot' codes, which is a poor interpretation on the codes alone.

Option D has interpreted 'oxygen negative' as 'devoid of oxygen', which could be correct but it has not used the code 'hot opposite hot' as 'hot and cold' and in turn 'temperatures'. Instead it has used the code 'hot'.

Question 19

Answer and rationale

506T, 901, 902, 903, 904, 905, U, UT, YTY, ▲ X

The code combines the words 'aliens opposite', 'warm', 'sociable', 'aggression', 'tense', 'cynical', 'negative', 'negative opposite', 'slow opposite slow', 'Mars enlarge'.

Option C 'The movement of the planets has a positive or negative impact on human characteristics' is the correct answer as it uses all the codes. 'Slow opposite' becomes 'fast' and when combined with 'slow' this becomes movement. 'Mars enlarge' becomes 'planets', 'negative opposite' becomes 'positive' and the codes 'warm', 'sociable', 'aggression', 'tense' and 'cynical' are combined to become 'characteristics'. The word 'impact' is added and this is an instance where you are being asked to make a more subtle judgement when a code appears to be missing. It is necessary to consider carefully all the options before determining that this is the correct one.

Option A has not used the combined codes of 'slow opposite' (fast) and 'slow' to become movement. In addition the code 'enlarge Mars' has not been applied, neither have the codes 'negative' and 'negative opposite'. The word 'influenced' has been introduced which cannot be correct due to the other missing codes.

Option B has not used the combined codes of 'slow opposite' (fast) and 'slow' to become movement. In addition the code 'enlarge Mars' has not been applied. The code 'aliens' has been introduced along with other words, which cannot be correct due to the other missing codes.

Option D has applied 'opposite' to characteristics and has also omitted the codes of 'movement', negative and positive. In addition the code 'enlarge Mars' has not been applied.

Option E has not used the code 'slow' but would need to be considered carefully as, otherwise, it could be a plausible interpretation.

Question 20

Answer and rationale

Options B and D 'tired' and 'narrow' would be the **two** most useful additions to the codes when attempting to convey the message 'The cold, thin air on Jupiter makes me very sleepy', the word 'narrow' being used for 'thin' and the word 'tired' being used for 'sleepy'. The other words in the message can be extrapolated from existing codes.

Option A 'planet' is not needed because 'Jupiter' could be extrapolated from Z ▲ 'similar Mars'.

Option C 'chilly' is not needed because 'cold' could be extrapolated from T W 'opposite hot'.

Option E 'atmosphere' is not needed because 'air' could be extrapolated from Z ◆ 'similar oxygen'.

Question 21

Answer and rationale

X V(903, 904), 🏃, 506, V(🏃☆), 502, □

The code combines the words 'enlarge unite aggression tense', 'me', 'aliens', 'unite me others', 'damage', 'home'.

Option C 'It makes me very hostile when aliens attack our planet' is the correct answer as it uses all the codes with, 'enlarge unite aggression tense' being used as 'very hostile', 'me' being used as 'I', 'unite me others' being used as 'our', 'damage' being used as 'attack' and 'home' being used as 'planet'.

Option A has failed to use 'unite aggression tense' as 'hostile'.

Option B has not used the code 'aliens'.

Option D has not used the code 'me' as 'I' or the code 'unite me others' as 'our'.

Option E has failed to use 'unite aggression tense' as 'hostile' and has omitted the code 'unite me others' as 'our'.

Question 22

Answer and rationale
Option E would be the best way to encode the message 'The fire damage to the warp drive is a very tense situation for us'.

⚱V☆, ♥, 502, 904X, 501

This option has the correct codes by using ⚱V☆ 'me unite others' as 'us', and 904X 'tense enlarge' as 'very tense', and 501 'warp' as 'warp drive'.

Option A has used the code for 'aliens' instead of the code for 'warp'.

Option B is the same as Option A but ordered differently.

Option C has not 'enlarged' tense to 'very tense'.

Option D has missed the code V 'unite' between 'me others' to form 'us'.

Question 23

Answer and rationale
→, X♥, XT902, 506, V(⚱☆)

The code combines the words 'ship', 'enlarge fire', 'enlarge opposite sociable', 'aliens', 'unite me others'.

Option A 'The aliens were very unfriendly and fired at our ship' is the correct answer as it uses all the codes with, 'enlarge fire' being used as 'fired', 'enlarge opposite sociable' being used as 'very unfriendly', 'unite me others' being used as 'our'.

Option B has failed to interpret 'enlarge fire' as 'fired' and has omitted the code 'enlarge opposite sociable' as 'very unfriendly'.

Option C has not 'enlarged' unfriendly to 'very unfriendly' and has used 'unite me others' as 'we'.

Option D has not used the code 'unite me others' as 'our'.

Option E has not used the code 'aliens' and has failed to interpret 'enlarge opposite sociable' as 'very unfriendly'.

Question 24

Answer and rationale

Option D would be the best way to encode the message 'Martians have the capacity to be both friendly and aggressive just like us.'

503, ▲506, V(902 903), V(⚤), Z

This option has the correct codes by using ▲506 'Mars aliens' as 'Martians', V(902 903) 'unite sociable aggression' as 'both friendly and aggressive', V(⚤) 'unite me others' as 'us' and Z 'similar' as 'just like'.

Option A has omitted the V to 'unite sociable aggression'.

Option B has failed to combine 'Mars' and 'aliens' as 'Martians' and has omitted to combine 'me' with 'others' to form 'us'.

Option C has omitted the code 'capacity'.

Option E has replaced the code 'capacity' with the code 'prefer'.

Question 25

Answer and rationale

V(Z♣ ♥), ☆, →, ■X, 501

The code combines the words 'unite similar hydrogen oxygen', 'others', 'ship', 'heavy enlarge' and 'warp'.

Option B 'Some gases are heavier than others and affect the ship's speed' is the correct answer as it uses all the codes, with 'unite similar hydrogen oxygen' being used as 'some gases', 'heavy enlarge' being used as 'heavier' and 'warp' being used as speed.

Option A has failed to interpret 'unite similar hydrogen oxygen' as 'some gases' and has not used 'warp' as 'speed'.

Option C has repeated the code 'warp' by using it as both 'warp' and 'speed'.

Option D has used the code 'unite similar hydrogen oxygen' as both 'gases' and 'like oxygen and hydrogen'.

Option E has failed to use the codes 'others' and 'heavy enlarge'.

Question 26

Answer and rationale

Options C and E 'bounces' and 'colours' would be the **two** most useful additions to the codes when attempting to convey the message 'The red and orange glow from Mars reflects off our ship'. The word 'bounces' could be used for 'reflects off' and the word 'colours' could stand for 'red and yellow'. The other words in the message can be extrapolated from existing codes or are irrelevant.

Option A 'mirror' could be used for 'reflects' but it would not convey 'reflects off' as well as 'bounces'.

Option B 'ember' could be used for 'glow' but we could already extrapolate 'glow' from 'hot'.

Option D 'shine' could be used for 'reflects' but it would not convey 'reflects off' as well as 'bounces'.

Chapter 12
The Non-Cognitive Analysis subtest

This chapter will help you to:

- understand the purpose and the format of the Non-Cognitive Analysis subtest;
- prepare for the Non-Cognitive Analysis subtest using examples of non-cognitive analysis questions;
- encourage the best approach when answering non-cognitive analysis questions.

Introduction

In 2011 the UKCAT Consortium decided that candidates would not be required to take the Non-Cognitive Analysis subtest (the behavioural test). However, the Consortium have stated on their website that this test '… will be reintroduced into future years of testing after further research has taken place on the use of these scores.' As a result of this action consideration was given to the removal of the chapter but it was decided to retain it because the date of reintroduction of the behavioural test is not known.

Pearson VUE describes the purpose of this subtest as follows.

The Non-Cognitive Analysis subtest assesses aspects of a candidate's empathy, integrity, honesty or robustness. Some questions will describe situations where candidates have to decide what to do according to their opinions or values. There are no right or wrong answers. Rather, candidates are asked to choose an answer from a series of options that most closely reflects their value system and what they believe is appropriate in each situation. Other questions cover a range of behaviours, attitudes, experiences, reactions to stress and feelings of well-being. Some of the questions are specifically designed to measure the degree of honesty with which the questionnaire has been approached.

What are non-cognitive analysis tests?

The UKCAT Non-Cognitive Analysis subtest is basically a measure of an individual's personality in terms of their most likely traits (characteristics). Personality tests are generally formatted along similar lines in that they contain a range of statements that are rated according to one's own preferences, values and beliefs. They usually contain randomly mixed statements which load onto particular scales of personality, for example, ten statements that would all load onto your level of 'anxiety', or ten statements that would all load onto your level of 'empathy'. The robustness of these types of questionnaires is often dependent on having sufficient items for each scale; this will be discussed later in terms of the reliability and validity of these measures. It is not clear how many items and scales are actually contained in the UKCAT Non-Cognitive Analysis subtest. There are a large number of personality questionnaires available on the market; however, the majority are restricted to those who have been trained to use them.

The use of personality questionnaires in the commercial world as an aid to the recruitment, selection and development of staff has grown phenomenally over the last 20 years. Increasingly, organisations have realised that the levels of performance of staff with identical qualifications and skills differ greatly according to their 'personalities'. The consortium of universities using the UKCAT have introduced this type of assessment as an attempt to identify additional attributes and characteristics that it is believed do contribute to success in either medicine or dentistry careers; robustness, empathy and integrity.

The reliability and validity of personality questionnaires are limited. Test publishers should rigorously assess their questionnaires in order to arrive at a set of questions that best measure the intended scales (reliability) and these should then be validated against other measures of the same scales and, more importantly, external measures. For example, does your scale of integrity really relate to the level of integrity a person demonstrates in reality? In practice, the most rigorous measures available are not that great at actually predicting performance. For example, the very best measures of the scale of 'anxiety or stress' will only account for approximately 4 to 6 per cent of variability in an individual's actual level of stress. Therefore, there is up to a massive 96 per cent not accounted for by the personality test. A major factor here is that the very best of these types of tests are measuring an individual's likely personality traits but they do not measure their behaviour. For example, an individual who has high anxiety on a personality measure may not suffer from stress. Indeed, they may be highly driven to work long and hard, perhaps at some expense to their well-being but not necessarily.

The best professional use of these types of questionnaires is usually where they are used as a tool to elicit further information from a candidate regarding real-world evidence of their behaviours. Alternatively, they may be used as a very small part of a decision-making process alongside other information such as personal statements or testimonials, etc. It is to be expected or hoped that the information from the UKCAT Non-Cognitive Analysis subtest will be used in one of these ways.

According to the UKCAT website the results from the Non-Cognitive Analysis subtest will be in the form of a band from 'A' to 'E' as this reflects the nature of the questions. It is assumed that 'A' will represent a very high level of robustness, empathy and integrity, through to 'E' representing a very low level of these attributes.

If you are interested to learn more you can access more information about personality testing by looking up 'personality tests' on www.en.wikipedia.org.

Non-Cognitive Analysis subtest

The Non-Cognitive Analysis subtest is an onscreen test consisting of a series of questions which will take no longer than 30 minutes to complete. The actual number of questions is not given on the UKCAT website but generally this type of 'personality' questionnaire would contain somewhere between 100 and 160 questions in the given timescale. This is only an estimate and the actual number of questions may be fewer. This subtest differs from the other four UKCAT subtests in that there are **no right or wrong answers.**

Response formats and example questions

Some questions will be based around a piece of text followed by statements with which you will be asked to rate your level of agreement or disagreement. Some questions will present statements of how you might behave or think in certain situations, and general statements about how you may feel about others. You will be asked to rate the truth or falsity of these statements according to your own beliefs and values. Some questions will present paired statements that represent opposing points of view and you will be asked to indicate your level of agreement on a scale between the two statements. The example questions on the UKCAT website (www.ukcat.ac.uk) will provide a useful taster of the format of the questions.

Example questions

The following examples are intended to provide a sample of the types of questions that will be asked. They will be followed by an explanation of which trait/characteristic they are attempting to assess (these will only be capsule descriptions). Most of the questions will be measuring a bi-polar scale, for example, 'low anxiety' as opposed to 'high anxiety'. It should be noted that both ends of each scale can have advantages and disadvantages given the demands of situations. As a 'lay person' in the field of personality assessment you may not always be able to link questions in this way and it is advised that you do not spend time pondering this when you sit the UKCAT.

Unlike the other four subtests it will be of no value to you to provide a set of scored practice items. However, the section following this one will provide you with useful tips on how to approach this type of questionnaire.

Example 1

False	Somewhat False	Somewhat True	True

I know I can do things better than most people.

This type of question is attempting to measure your level of self-esteem – a 'False' response would load onto low self-esteem and a 'True' response would load onto high self-esteem with moderators between.

People with high self-esteem are confident in themselves and their abilities while low scorers lack confidence and believe that they are prone to failure. Conversely, high scorers may appear to be overconfident while low scorers may strive to do things better.

Example 2

False	Somewhat False	Somewhat True	True

I seem to have more bad luck than other people.

This type of question is attempting to measure your level of optimism – a 'False' response would load onto optimism and a 'True' response would load onto pessimism with moderators between.

Optimists are generally happy and cheerful and look to positive outcomes while pessimists can be gloomy or depressed and have a belief that fate dictates their future. Conversely, optimists may overlook some problems while pessimists may always be on the look out for what could go wrong.

Example 3

Strongly Agree	Agree	Disagree	Strongly Disagree

Are you easily annoyed if things don't go according to plan?

This type of question is attempting to measure your level of anxiety – a 'Strongly Agree' response would load onto high anxiety and a 'Strongly Disagree' response would load onto low anxiety with moderators between.

High scorers get frustrated when things go wrong and may worry or get stressed unnecessarily while low scorers are laid back and calm and do not have irrational fears. Conversely, high scorers may be extremely driven while low scorers may appear complacent.

Example 4

| Strongly Agree | Agree | Disagree | Strongly Disagree |

I would never lie or cheat even if the stakes were high.

This type of question is attempting to measure your level of what is often termed 'social desirability' or 'faking good or bad'. These types of scales are often used to indicate your level of honesty when completing the questionnaire – a 'Strongly Agree' response would load onto faking good and a 'Strongly Disagree' response would load onto faking bad with moderators between. This type of question often appears to be a trick question, which may lead one to believe that they should say that they never lie or cheat, but how realistic is this?

High 'faking good' may suggest that you have presented an unrealistic positive image of yourself while 'faking bad' may suggest that you have undesirable social habits. Conversely, someone with a high faking good score may really believe that they are more socially desirable than most even if this is unrealistic, while someone faking bad may really believe that they should admit to human failings.

Example 5

The following item would require you to indicate your position on the scale between the two statements.

I hardly ever meet problems or tasks that I can't easily overcome or complete.

-
-
-
-
-

I often meet problems or tasks that I find difficult to overcome or complete.

This type of question is attempting to measure your level of self-reliance or robustness – a response closer to the top statement would load onto robustness and a response towards the bottom statement would load onto a sensitivity/fragility with moderators between.

Robustness would suggest a capability to deal with almost any eventuality while sensitivity would suggest that some situations would be too overwhelming. Conversely, robustness may make someone appear to be to hard-headed and task focused while sensitivity may indicate a more tender-minded, intuitive approach.

If you want to complete a Non-Cognitive Analysis subtest, a full subtest is provided in the Questions companion book *Practice Test, Questions and Answers for the UKCAT*, © Rosalie Hutton and Glenn Hutton, 2010. Learning Matters Ltd.

Best approach when answering the Non-Cognitive Analysis subtest

- Answer the questions as honestly as possible. There may not always be sufficient information but answer the best you can.

- Answer all the questions as they will all load onto the scales being measured (other than items that they may be trialling but you will not know which these are).

- Be spontaneous. Your first response is usually a more accurate reflection of how you really feel.

- Do not try to give the answers that you think are correct as this may produce a profile that is completely different to how you really see yourself.

- When answering questions that appear to be assessing integrity, be realistic – these types of questions are often designed to load onto a scale that would suggest that you are attempting to present a more positive image of yourself than is realistic.

- Do not spend time pondering items by trying to second guess what they might be measuring.

- Do not try to answer from a particular scenario – for example, how you are with your close friends as compared to how you are at work. Just give your most natural and spontaneous response.

- Remember, you cannot cheat on this type of test; the result would be a profile that is not you and if higher levels of certain characteristics are deemed important in medicine and you do not possess them then maybe it would be an unsuitable career for you (this statement is of course subject to the comments made previously on reliability and validity and the use of the information).

Part III
Preparing for the BioMedical Admissions Test (BMAT)

The following chapters will help you to:

- understand the purpose and the format of the BioMedical Admissions Test (BMAT);
- understand the different sections and how to tackle them;
- prepare for the test using BMAT-style questions.

The BioMedical Admissions Test (BMAT) was designed to help admissions officers cope with the problem of rising standards among medical school and veterinary school applicants. By examining the skills required to succeed in medicine and veterinary science, such as the application of scientific knowledge, decision-making and logical argument, they can differentiate better on paper between candidates who have the same top A1 grades.

The BMAT has always generated a lot of anxiety among students who are usually unsure of the standard and importance of the test. Now it has been joined in the admissions process by its friend the UKCAT, its purpose may seem more unclear than before, especially as only a handful of UK medical and veterinary schools require it for entry to their courses (see Table 1). The first step to performing well in the BMAT is to understand its purpose and format. Then you can progress to familiarising yourself with the format of questions used and, finally, attempt practice questions and tests to build your confidence.

Whether you're reading this part of the book in a state of panic a week before the test or as a primer to familiarise yourself with the test, if you follow the advice given here you will not only alleviate a lot of your anxiety but will also pick up those extra crucial marks that can make all the difference to the success of your university application.

Table 1 Courses requiring BMAT

Institution	UCAS	Institution code
University of Cambridge	C05	A100, A101, D100
Imperial College London	I50	A100, B900, B9N2
Oxford University	O33	A100, BC98
Royal Veterinary College	R84	D100, D101, D102
University College London	U80	A100

Important note: if you are also applying to universities that require you to sit the UKCAT, you must sit this in addition to the BMAT exam.

Understanding the BMAT layout and scoring

The BMAT test has three parts and is two hours long in total.

Section 1	Aptitude and Skills	1 hour
Section 2	Scientific Knowledge and Applications	30 minutes
Section 3	Writing Task	30 minutes

These are all examined at the same time, but on separate answer sheets and with separate timings – hence you cannot run over on one part and make it up on another. Think of them as three separate exams taken during the same sitting.

Sections 1 and 2 are multiple choice or single best answer and will be marked by a computer. Some of you may not have met this style of answer sheet before, so it is important to familiarise yourself with it before the exam (visit the BMAT website at www.admissionstests.cambridgeassessment.org.uk) so that you can appreciate the importance of recording the right answer in the right space. This may sound obvious but every year students miss out a question without leaving the correct space for it blank on their answer sheets. Only later do they realise what they have done, which inevitably leads to extra stress and mistakes.

Use an HB pencil for your answers (the propelling variety is good) and try not to rub out. If you do make a mistake, rub out your answer completely before you fill in your new answer. If you do not, the computer will read any remaining traces of your first answer and will assume you have chosen two solutions, thus invalidating that answer. This style of multiple-choice assessment is becoming increasingly popular among medical and veterinary schools, so it is as well to get used to the format now.

For Section 3 ('Writing Task'), use a pen and write neatly. Watch your spelling and punctuation – there are marks for these and it would be silly to throw away marks on simple points like this.

How the BMAT is marked

For Section 1 ('Aptitude and Skills') and Section 2 ('Scientific Knowledge and Applications'), BMAT converts your marks into a score reported to the nearest decimal point on a nine-point BMAT scale.

For Section 3 ('Writing Task'), your paper will be marked for content on a scale of 0–5, and a score for written English on a scale of A, C, E. Each essay is double marked and, if the mark is the same or a single point in difference, then the average is given. If there is a larger difference in marks, then it is marked for a third time. Obviously this is rather labour intensive for the BMAT examiners, but they do it to ensure that the marks are objective and that you won't be marked down just because one examiner doesn't agree with your arguments. A copy of your essay is sent to the institutions you applied to, and they often use it for discussion in your interview. (They will give you a copy beforehand.)

An important point to note here is that, unlike A-levels or GCSEs, you are very unlikely to score full marks on the BMAT. Figures 1, 2 and 3 show the scores from the 2010 BMAT students. As you can see, they follow a normal distribution, with very high scores being rare and low scores being even rarer. Please remember that, however badly you think you will do on the test, it is almost impossible to 'fail' the BMAT – the test has been designed so that the average candidate for medicine, such as yourself, will score around 5.0.

Figure 1 BMAT Section 1 scores 2010

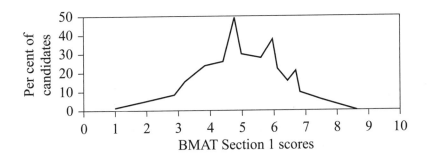

Figure 2 BMAT Section 2 scores 2010

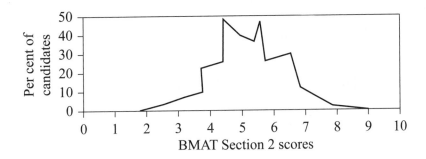

The BMAT examiners know that only a few very exceptional applicants will score higher than 7.0, and that 6.0 represents a comparatively high score. There is, therefore, no need to panic if you find the exam difficult because it is more than likely that most other candidates will find it just as difficult. Some students do better on one section than on another, and it is for this reason that BMAT provides a breakdown of your scores so that your assessors can get a good idea of what your strengths and weaknesses are, rather than an overall average score that does not provide them with as much information. A downside of this, however, is that you cannot spend lots of time practising one part of the test in the hope that it will boost your mark; you need to prepare for all the sections of the test to the same standard.

Figure 3 BMAT Section 3 scores 2010

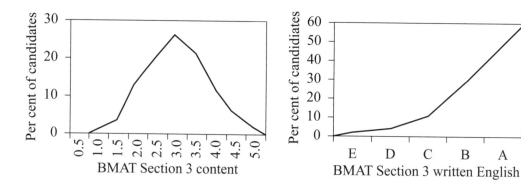

As you can see from the above graphs, most candidates score either 'A' or 'B' for written English, although if this is something you have difficulty with it is worth paying attention to.

The scores for context are more widely spread, with the majority of candidates scoring between 2.0 and 4.0. A small amount of preparation for Section 3 to increase your mark by 1 point will therefore increase your chances of scoring in the top percentage of your year group. More details of the criteria for awarding each score are available on the BMAT website.

How your BMAT scores will be used

How your BMAT scores will be used varies between universities. Some place a lot of weight on BMAT scores and use them as a criterion for inviting candidates for interview. Others use the BMAT as just one part of the application process, giving weight also to your personal statement, A1 scores and UCAS form when deciding whether or not to invite you to interview and offer you a place. So the BMAT is important, but don't prepare excessively for it at the expense of working on your A2s. If you get your UCAS form completed by the end of September, you will have a whole month to prepare for the BMAT.

If you are unclear as to how important your BMAT score will be for your application, check out the details in the prospectus or email the applications officer at your prospective university. If you do this before you sit the test you can, first, make sure you prepare appropriately and, secondly, will save yourself a great deal of angst and worry if you think you have done badly on the day. The timescale for applying to sit the BMAT exam is detailed below. Check with your school or college if you are at all unsure about the arrangements.

BMAT application process: key dates for 2012

These dates are as listed by BMAT. Check their website regularly for any changes to the schedule.

1 October 2012
Closing date for entries.

15 October 2012
Closing date for late entries (fees payable)

7 November 2012
BMAT test

21 November 2012
Results released via Results Online system.

The fee for 2012 is £42.50 in the UK and £72.50 for international candidates. Late entry fee is £30 extra. (This may seem a lot, but it's cheaper than the UKCAT.) You will need to be entered by your school or college and you must check that they can administer the test for you – let them know well before the end of August that you want to be entered for the test. Some schools and colleges have combined sittings, so you should check where you are meant to be sitting the test in advance of the day itself. If you have left school or college, you can make an application to sit the test at one of the open centres listed on the BMAT website.

In the following chapters the three sections of the BMAT test are examined in detail, with advice, worked answers and practice papers to test yourself. Don't try to work through the whole test in one sitting: work on each section of the test independently, in conjunction with the sample and past papers available on the BMAT website, until you are confident that you know how to tackle the type of questions you will meet in the real test. Familiarising yourself with the type and format of the questions and practising how to solve them are absolutely the best preparation you can do.

Chapter 13
Section 1: Aptitude and Skills

35 marks/60 minutes
Multiple choice or single best answer
No calculators allowed

During your time at university you will rely heavily on problem-solving skills, reasoning and analytical thinking in order to progress with your studies and to deal with the new ideas and concepts that you will meet. This is what Section 1 is for: it is attempting to find out if you have these necessary skills to cope with an undergraduate course in medicine, dentistry or veterinary science. So, although a lot of the questions may seem unrelated to what you have been studying in your A1 and A2 courses, the underlying skills needed to answer them correctly are very important.

You may be panicking because you think you don't have these necessary skills, or you may have heard that you can't practise for the test because you've either 'got it' or you haven't. BMAT itself says that 'An approach to developing these thinking skills can be taught, and the skills will improve with familiarity and practice. We encourage this because we think these skills are really worthwhile: they are useful skills in many walks of life, and very important for success in higher education.' So if you really want that university place and to do well once you get there, now is the time to invest some time in preparation.

BMAT goes on to say: 'What you cannot do is to be taught to answer as if you were a performing seal. There are no simple short cuts – you really do have to think the answers through.' While this is true to some extent, you can compare preparing for the BMAT with preparing for your GCSEs or A-levels. Normally, after you have finished studying the curriculum content, in order to pass the exam you work through practice and past papers. Doing the past papers won't teach you the knowledge or skills that you need to pass the exam, but familiarising yourself with the type of questions that are asked and figuring out how to apply your knowledge are vital parts of the preparation process.

This type of preparation is just what you should do for the BMAT. It is reassuring that the examiners themselves note there is no special 'trick' to answering questions: all the knowledge you require has been taught to you already at GCSE level. What you can do is get yourself up to speed by practising lots of BMAT-style questions so that, when you get into the exam, you can question-spot and recognise how questions should be solved.

Important note: on the BMAT website there is a list of recommended reading on how to improve your thinking skills. You may find such reading beneficial, but bear in mind that these books are pretty wordy and not that useful for practising for the BMAT, especially if you have limited time on your hands.

Section 1 is worth 35 marks and tests:

- problem solving (approx. 30 mins);
- understanding argument (approx. 15 mins);
- data analysis and inference (approx. 15 mins).

This means you have 60 minutes to get 35 marks (i.e. less than 2 minutes for each question). The marks tend to be split equally between the three question types, which are spread throughout the paper. However, the problem-solving questions take longer to read, so allow yourself a little extra time for these – but you will have to be speedy on the other types of questions.

There is no negative marking on the BMAT, so if you run short of time a guess is always better than no answer at all. For most of the multiple-choice questions you have at least a 20 per cent chance of getting it right. If you don't know an answer, fill in one answer as a guess and place a '?' by the side to come back to it later, if you have the time. Never leave an answer blank because you may run out of time at the end and thus never get the chance to make a guess at it.

However short of time you are, you must always read the question carefully. While the examiners do not set questions to catch you out deliberately, the questions often require you to perform a calculation and then give the remainder as the answer, or the questions may use different units from the answer choices. If you are rushing, you may not spot these nuances and all your calculations will go to waste. Also, beware of feeling relieved that the answer you have obtained is offered as a choice – the examiners also include the most commonly worked-out incorrect answers as possible solutions in the answer sets.

On the BMAT website you will find a number of practice papers you should do in exam conditions to get a feel for what's required of you. You can also visit www.ucl.ac.uk/lapt/bmat.htm. Here you will find lots of excellent logic and problem-solving questions that test the same skills used in the BMAT – they even talk you through the solutions. Attempt the answer yourself first and then either pat yourself on the back or see where you went wrong. Rather than sit down and do them all in one mammoth session, do a few a day – that way you'll be consolidating your learning. Note that some of the questions are the same as those on the BMAT website.

Below you will find worked examples of BMAT-style questions, with a step-by-step guide on how to approach them. After these you will find a BMAT-style test with answers and explanations of how to work them out. By working through these examples you should feel much more confident in your ability to tackle the BMAT.

Example: *data analysis*

1   The graph below shows how the flow rate of liquid out of a cylinder varies with time. The area marked *B* is twice as large as *A*. Which **two** of the following are false?

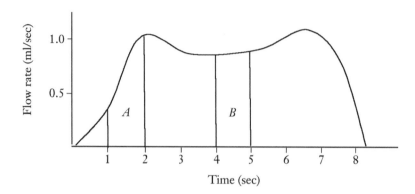

A   The rate of fluid flow after 4 seconds is twice what it is after 1 second.

B   The average rate of fluid flow is twice as great between 4 and 5 seconds, compared with 1 and 2 seconds.

C   The flow rate increases twice as rapidly between 4 and 5 seconds as it does between 3 and 4 seconds.

D   The amount of fluid flowing between 1 and 2 seconds is half as much as the amount flowing between 4 and 5 seconds.

How to solve it

First, work out what the graph is showing you – they even tell you: flow rate on the y axis, time on the x axis. Then, note that $B = 2 \times A$ (given) and realise that two of the possibilities are correct and that they want you to mark down the false answers. Don't be caught out! It is easiest to work out which ones are correct and then write down the other two.

A   The rate of fluid flow after 4 seconds is twice what it is after 1 second.
We're dealing with rate of fluid flow, so read from the y axis. The flow rate at 4 seconds is around 0.9 ml/s; the flow rate after 1 second is around 0.3 ml/s. Because 0.9 is not (2×0.3), this is false.

B   The average rate of fluid flow is twice as great between 4 and 5 seconds, compared with 1 and 2 seconds.

They have told you that the volume (area under the graph) of B is $2A$. The three variables described by the graph are time, flow rate and volume. The volume has doubled, whereas the time period (1 second) is constant. Therefore the flow rate increase must be double.

C   The flow rate increases twice as rapidly between 4 and 5 seconds as it does between 3 and 4 seconds.
The rate of flow is the graph line. It is flat between 3 and 4 seconds, and it's still flat between 4 and 5 seconds – i.e. the flow rate is remaining constant. Therefore this choice is false.

D   The amount of fluid flowing between 1 and 2 seconds is half as much as the amount flowing between 4 and 5 seconds.
The y axis is rate of flow, the x is time. Remember that 'Rate of flow = Volume/Time'. Thus the area under the graph is volume. This is why they told you that B was twice A. So D is correct.

B and D are correct. Therefore you have to mark down A and C on your form.

The lesson here is that, although the questions in themselves are not difficult, there are lots of easy mistakes you could make in the heat of the moment, especially when you are under time pressure. Force yourself always to read the questions carefully before you jump in and solve them: you will save yourself a lot of time and will avoid making mistakes.

Example: problem-solving

2   Mr Jones has to renew the white lines on a 1 km stretch of road. Each edge of the road is marked with a solid line and there is a 'dashed' line in the centre. Drivers are warned of approaching bends by two curved arrows. Mr Jones will have to paint four curved arrows. The manufacturers have printed the following guidance on each 5 litre drum of paint:

Solid lines – 5 metres per litre.
Dashed lines – 20 metres per litre.
Curved arrows – 3 litres each.

How many drums of paint will Mr Jones require?

A   53

B   92

C   93

D   103

E   462

How to solve it

The solid lines require 200 litres for each side of the road (1,000/5).
The dashed line requires 50 litres (1,000/20).
The arrows require 12 litres (3 × 4).
Total paint required is 462 litres (200 + 200 + 50 + 12).

Beware! Most candidates at this point will go for choice E. The question asks how many **drums** of paint you require – you have worked out the litres required.

Total drums required is 92.4 (462/5).

You will have to round up to nearest drum. Therefore C is correct.

All the choices given here will seem correct – if you calculate the answer incorrectly. As you become more efficient at answering the questions, you will find time to double-check your answers. If a question at first seems too easy, look for the hidden twist. For example, forgetting to round up the drums may lead you incorrectly to select B, or only having a solid line on one side of the road will lead you incorrectly to select A.

Example: understanding argument

3   Vegetarian food can be healthier than a traditional diet. Research has shown that vegetarians are less likely to suffer from heart disease and obesity than meat eaters. Concern has been expressed that vegetarians do not get enough protein in their diet, but it has been demonstrated that, by selecting foods carefully, vegetarians are able amply to meet their needs in this respect.

Which of the following best expresses the main conclusion of the above argument?

A   A vegetarian diet can be better for health than a traditional diet.

B   Adequate protein is available from a vegetarian diet.

C   A traditional diet is very high in protein.

D   A balanced diet is more important for health than any particular food.

E   Vegetarians are unlikely to suffer from heart disease and obesity.

How to solve it

These questions are tough, mainly because it takes quite some time to read the passage and the answers. The best way to approach this is to read the passage and then to pick holes in all the choices offered. Note that all the choices could be argued to be a conclusion – the question asks for the best choice (which is often the only one you can't pick a hole in). The conclusion is sometimes a statement in the text – although it needn't necessarily be at the end.

A A vegetarian diet can be better for health than a traditional diet.
   This is the first line of the passage – think of news reports, which always have their conclusions at the start. Hold this one in reserve for now.

B Adequate protein is available from a vegetarian diet.
   This is mentioned in the passage, but only by selecting foods carefully. It is doubtful if this is the main conclusion.

C A traditional diet is very high in protein.
   It may well be, but this is an inference from the passage – vegetarians don't get enough protein so meat eaters must do(?) This is not the main conclusion here.

D A balanced diet is more important for health than any particular food.
   It doesn't say so anywhere in the passage. Don't let what you know cloud your judgement about what the passage says. This is not the main conclusion.

E Vegetarians are unlikely to suffer from heart disease and obesity.
   Be careful! Vegetarians are *less* likely, not *un*likely! There could be a 98 per cent chance, which is still less likely than 99 per cent, but still very high. Not the conclusion.

So, there is a choice between A and B. If in doubt, always go for the statement that has been mentioned explicitly in the passage. This may seem rather simple and make you second-guess, but remember there is nothing subtle about the BMAT. The best answer is A.

Now, try the practice test for Section 1. Check your answers after you have completed the entire test. There are fewer questions in this test than in the actual BMAT exam. This is so you can take your time with each question and focus on how you are working out the answers rather than using an element of guesswork. Make sure you are definitely happy with each question before moving on. Also included are explanations of how the correct answers were reached so that you can gain an understanding of how to tackle the questions and also learn from your mistakes.

Section 1 practice test

1   Happy Pharma sells two types of cough medicine, which can be bulk-bought in mixed boxes.

24 Muco-eaze and 20 Tickle-gone costs £134.

20 Muco-eaze and 24 Tickle-gone costs £130.

What is the price of a single unit of Muco-eaze?

2   A dentist has appointments with 1,800 patients in a year. Twenty per cent of his patients are female, and 50 per cent of his male patients are over 60. He finds that, as a rule, one in 20 patients needs further dental work after they come for a routine check-up.

Assuming that all his patients attend for a routine check-up in a year, what is the number of male patients under the age of 60 who will need further dental work? Give your answer to the nearest whole number.

A   20

B   36

C   18

D   72

E   9

3   In the waiting room of the clinic, Tom places some toy-bricks in a pile. The red brick is above the blue brick, which is above the yellow brick. The green brick is below the blue brick and above the white brick.

The yellow brick must be:

A   Below the white, but above the red.

B   Above the blue, but not above the green.

C   Below the blue, but not necessarily below the red.

D   Below the blue, but not necessarily below the green.

4 Bob the plumber charges a flat call-out rate, plus a fixed fee per half hour of work, charged to each complete half hour.

Andy pays Bob £210 for $2\frac{1}{2}$ hours' work.

Brian pays Bob £150 for $1\frac{1}{2}$ hours' work.

How much will Clive pay for 1 hour of work?

5 At school sports day, Anthony finished the 5,000m race ahead of Ben, but after Charlie. Damian beat Charlie, but not Edward.

In what position did Damian finish?

A First

B Second

C Third

D Fourth

E Fifth

Questions 6 to 8 refer to the following information.

A blood transfusion laboratory audits 5,000 transfusion reactions and notes their causes, shown in the pie chart below:

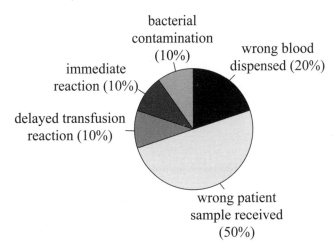

6 How many reactions were due to the wrong type of blood being dispensed?

7 After an awareness drive, the number of wrong patient samples received fell by 250. If all other categories remained constant, what percentage of the reactions is now caused by wrong patient samples? Give your answer to the nearest whole number.

8 If the number of transfusions given increases by 15%, what would be the predicted number of immediate transfusion reactions (based on original data)?

9 If you drink too much alcohol and have a hangover, you may have a headache or tremors. Some, but not all, hung-over people with a headache also have tremors. Some, but not all, hung-over people with tremors also have a headache.

Which one of the options, A to F, correctly lists the following statements in order of their probability, listing the least likely first?

1 Someone suffering from a hangover will have a headache.
2 Someone suffering from a hangover will have a headache and tremors.
3 Someone suffering from a hangover will have a headache or tremors.

A 1, 2, 3

B 1, 3, 2

C 2, 1, 3

D 2, 3, 1

E 3, 1, 2

F 3, 2, 1

10 Two nurses, Amelia and Boris, each collect blood samples from my patients on the ward and do their rounds hourly. They are both as hard working as each other and blood samples are ready to be collected all the time. Unfortunately I can never remember at what times they visit the ward, so I just give the blood samples to the first nurse who comes along. Strangely, I discover over the year that Amelia collects more blood from me than Boris.

Amelia visits the ward at a minutes past the hour, and Boris visits the ward at b minutes past the hour. If Amelia visits the ward in the first half of the hour, which **one** of the following would explain the higher probability of Amelia coming to the ward first?

A $b > 30$

B $0 < (b - a) < 30$

C $0 < (b - a) < 60$

D $a > b$

E $a/b < 1$

11 The spread of HIV-AIDS is a subject which should greatly concern the human race. The march of this disease through our populations should be checked before it is too late. Our future as a species depends on the continued research and investigation into finding a cure, and we should not take comfort from the limited success of antiretroviral drugs. We should all give generously to charities which support research into this deadly disease in order to protect the future of our children.

Which of the following is closest to the underlying assumption in the passage above?

A   HIV-AIDS is incurable.

B   Antiretroviral drugs are ineffective.

C   Donating to charity can help to cure HIV-AIDS.

D   Charities provide most of the funding for HIV-AIDS research.

12 On Paige ward there are 20 nurses. They must all complete at least one training module in a year, but no more than four.

Each of the four modules has to be completed before moving onto the next one, in a sequential process (e.g. 1 → 2 → 3 → 4). Thirty-six modules are taken in total.

1 nurse takes module 4.

5 nurses take module 3.

How many nurses complete module 2?

A   4

B   5

C   9

D   10

E   15

13 There are 40 students in year 12, and all take biology.
75% of students study biology only.
50% study chemistry, and 75% study maths.
5% of students study all three subjects, and 20% study either maths or chemistry.

If 5 students study biology and maths only, how many study biology and chemistry, but not maths?

A   2

B   3

C   4

D   5

Questions 14 to 17 refer to the following article.

Is bleach to blame for childhood asthma?

In a paper published this month, a group from Bristol University demonstrate a link between childhood exposure to domestic cleaning products and the development of persistent wheeze in children; a condition which often progresses to asthma. The study followed a cohort of more than 7,000 children until the age of 3.5 as part of the Avon Longitudinal Study of Parents and Children (ALSPAC). Analysis of questionnaires delivered both during and after pregnancy formed the basis of the study, with mothers being asked a number of questions regarding health and lifestyle choices. The participants were asked how often they used common household chemicals such as bleach, disinfectant, air-freshener and cleaning products, with their responses quantified to create a quotient of total chemical burden (TCB). The analysis suggested that no single product was solely implicated in the association with infant wheezing, and the authors were not able to determine whether the observed effect was due to in utero or postnatal exposure. However, given the strong correlation between prenatal and postnatal TCB scores found, and their association with persistent wheezing, it is likely that this represents postnatal exposure with a direct inflammatory insult to the airways (rather than a prenatal priming of airway inflammation in response to postnatal exposures such as airborne allergens). The headlines therefore centre on the statistically significant link between postnatal exposure to domestic chemical products and persistent wheezing illness in young children up to the age of 3.5 years, supporting an effect on the development of airway inflammation and asthma rather than a fundamental effect on airway development in utero.

With the incidence of asthma continuing to rise (the number of sufferers has tripled between 1970 and 2000), there has been much interest in the role environmental factors may play in causing asthma. Much speculation has centred on a possible link between household chemicals and asthma, especially given that the market for household cleaners has grown in line with the increased prevalence of the disease, and the observation that people, especially mothers with young children, spend most of the day indoors. However, the Avon analysis is at odds with a similar study, published in 2003 which found no association between direct exposure to domestic volatile organic compounds and wheezing illness in children aged 9–11. In defence, the authors of the Avon study speculate that in this age category 'the majority of wheezing illness is likely to be established asthma and this may have a different aetiology to wheezing illnesses that develop in early childhood'. Another consideration is that, whereas previous observational studies have consistently identified a link between chemical exposure and asthma, few interventional studies have been able to document such an association. This may be due to participant numbers, duration of exposure or, most significantly, the observed association in observational studies could be confounded by a factor which is a determinant of asthma and is also associated with exposure to volatile organic compounds.

Such a confounding factor may be cleanliness itself. A popular explanation for the increasing incidence of autoimmune diseases in childhood cites the underexposure of children to environmental antigens whilst their immune systems are developing, so that they later develop diseases of atopy. Proponents of this theory cite observations that the increased incidence of asthma has followed the spread of urbanisation from the north southwards, and no doubt could interpret the results of the Avon study to confirm that a hyper-clean environment causes asthma. While these considerations could be integrated into the relationship between chemicals and childhood wheeze, critics point to countries such as Hong Kong, Sweden and Thailand, which have comparable levels of domestic cleaner usage and yet have the lowest rates of severe childhood wheeze. In a statement Professor Andrew Peacock, of the British Thoracic Society, said: 'More long-term studies are needed before we advise pregnant women to throw out all their air fresheners.'

Answer the following questions, assuming the information in the article is accurate.

14 Which one of the following statements can we safely conclude to be accurate?

A Being too clean causes asthma.

B There are more asthma sufferers today than there were 30 years ago.

C It is likely that just one product will be found to cause childhood wheezing.

D Exposure to cleaning products in utero is more damaging than post-natal exposure.

15 The main message of the article is that:

A Asthma is a dangerous disease in childhood.

B There is a strong link between cleaning product use and the development of wheezing.

C It is not possible to identify a cause-and-effect relationship between any factor and asthma.

D Pregnant women should take care to avoid exposure to cleaning products.

16 If 10,000 people suffered from asthma in 1970, and the rate of increase mentioned in the article stays constant, how many sufferers will there be in 2030?

A 30,000

B 60,000

C 90,000

D 120,000

E 150,000

17 Which one of the following is not expressly mentioned by the article?

A Hong Kong, Sweden and Thailand have the lowest rates of severe childhood wheeze.

B There is much interest in the role environmental factors play in causing asthma.

C The market for household cleaners has grown in line with the increased prevalence of asthma.

D Children in the age group 9–11 suffer only from established asthma.

E Previous observational studies have identified a link between chemical exposure and asthma.

18 Damian test drives a variety of cars and measures their speed at 50 seconds from a standing start. Their profiles are shown below.

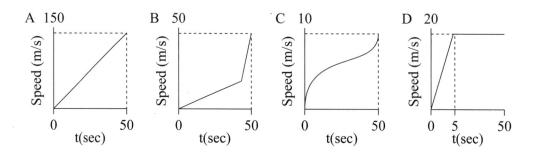

Put the cars in order of speed of acceleration:

A abcd

B bcda

C cabd

D dabc

E adbc

19 £400 in a will is divided among five charities. The will states that no two charities are to get the same amount of money, and each is to have at least £20. The donations are to be given out according to the charity's size: the largest gets the most, the smallest the least. If these rules are adhered to, what is the largest donation that the third biggest charity can receive?

A 22

B 120

C 119

D 118

E 121

Questions 20 to 22 refer to the following information.

A medical school has student dormitories on both sides of its campus. The girls' dormitories are on the south side and the boys' dormitories are on the north side. Because of student protests, the Dean decides to integrate the dormitories and to move the first student on the alphabetical list, Miss Adams, from the south side to the north side.

The registry list of room, rent and test scores (before the move) is shown below.

South side (girls)			North side (boys)		
Student surname	Rent paid (£)	Test score	Student surname	Rent paid (£)	Test score
Adams	80	140	Hill	65	130
Brown	100	120	Ibrahim	70	145
Cowen	55	130	Jones	110	125
Docker	60	125	Kent	95	140
Evans	35	130	Long	75	120
Fetts	40	120	McNamara	70	125
Gower	50	145	Norman	85	130
Total	**420**	**910**		**570**	**915**

20 What is the average rent paid (to the nearest whole number) on the south side of the campus after Miss Adams' move?

A 56

B 57

C 58

D 59

21 By how much will the average test score on the north side of the campus rise after Miss Adams moves? Give your answer to the nearest whole number.

A 0

B 1

C 2

D 3

22 If all the rents rise by 7.5% next year, what will the total rent bill be?

A £990

B £1,039.50

C £1064.25

D £1,089

23 A wine stopper is made of aluminium with a density of $2.0 g/cm^3$. Its dimensions are shown below.

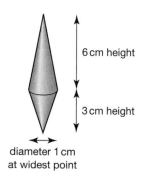

6 cm height

3 cm height

diameter 1 cm
at widest point

What is the mass of the wine stopper if the volume of a cone is described by $\frac{1}{3}\pi r^2 h$? Give your answer as a value of π.

END OF TEST

Section 1 practice test: answers

Question number	Correct response	Comments	Marks
1	£3.50		1
2	B		1
3	D		1
4	£120		1
5	B		1
6	1,000		1
7	47%		1
8	575		1
9	C		1
10	B		1
11	C		1
12	D		1
13	B		1
14	B	If plus any other answer, no mark	1
15	C		1
16	C		1
17	D		1
18	D		1
19	D		1
20	B		1
21	B		1
22	C		1
23	1.5π		1

Section 1 practice test: explanation of answers

1 Happy Pharma: £3.50

Muco-eaze = x, Tickle-gone = y

A. $24x + 20y = 134$
B. $20x + 24y = 130$

$a - b = 4x - 4y = 4$

$$\therefore x = 1 + y$$

a. $24(1 + y) + 20y = 134$ b. $20x + (24 \times 2.5) = 130$
   $24 + 24y + 20y = 134$ $20x = 70$
            $44y = 110$ $x = 3.5$
              $y = 2.5$

Check in a: $84 + 50 = 134$

$\therefore$ Muco-eaze = £3.50.

2 Dentist and his patients: B
1,800 patients, 20% female (thus 80% male); 50% male patients are over 60 (thus 50% of 80% of 1,800 patients are under 60); 1/20 consult; $1,440 \times 0.5 \times 1/20 = 36$.

3 Tom and his bricks: D
The only way to do this one is by a diagram. Once you have done this, it is clear that the only possible answer is D.

Possible combinations:

```
R   R   R
B   B   B
Y   G   G
G   Y   W
W   W   Y
```

4 Bob the plumber: £120.

Andy $x + 5y = 210$
Brian $x + 3y = 150$

$A - B: 2y = 60 \therefore$ each half hour = £30

Clive pays $60 + (2 \times 30) = £120$.

5 School sports day: B

A diagram helps:

ⒺDamian did not beat Edward.

Ⓓ

Damian beat Charlie.

Ⓒ

Anthony finished after Charlie.

Ⓐ

Anthony finished ahead of Ben.

Ⓑ

Blood bank (6–8)

6 1000
20% of 5000

7 47%
Wrong patient = 2500 – 250 = 2250
2250/4750 = 47.4 = 47%.

8 575
New number of transfusions = 5750
10% = 575.

9 Hangovers and headaches: C (2, 1, 3)
'Or' is more probable than specific illness, which in turn is more probable than 'and'.
Watch that you list them in the correct order (i.e. and<specific<or).

10 Amelia and Boris: B
There is a lot of wording in this question, but many of the statements allow you to
eliminate the given answer choices. Note that a and b are probabilities relating to
Amelia and Boris.

A This choice does not explain why Amelia should come first as it is stated that blood
samples become available at all times (i.e. not just in the first half of the hour).

B This choice is correct. Imagine Amelia comes at 29 minutes past (so within the
first half of the hour, as stated). In order for B to be fulfilled, Boris must visit the
ward between 30 and 58 minutes past (note the < symbol is used, not ⩽) i.e.
Amelia will always come first.

C Although this choice also describes the time condition as in B, it will not explain
why Amelia comes first. If we use the example time for Amelia as in B (a = 29), the
value of b could be anything between 30 and 88. Any value >60 would mean Boris
visited the ward before Amelia, because the difference in minutes would mean he
visits in the next hour, before Amelia.

D A lot of people will choose this one because it seems to describe that Amelia
comes before Boris. However, the probability of Amelia and Boris visiting the
ward is stated to be the same; what we are trying to find out is a description of
why Amelia comes first (i.e. a condition of time).

E The same explanation as above holds for this answer; the probability of visiting
the ward is actually $a = b$.

11 HIV-AIDS: C

The clue is in the last sentence when it says 'we should all give generously to charities... to protect the future of our children'. Thus it's therefore assuming that this money will help cure HIV-AIDS. The others aren't that convincing either. With this type of question, if you cannot decide between two answers, always go with your original 'hunch': experience shows that it is generally correct.

12 Nurses and training: D

			Modules
1		10	10
1 + 2	c	5	10
1 + 2 + 3	b	4	12
1 + 2 + 3 + 4	a	1	4
			36

It is easiest to draw a table.

1 nurse takes module 4, so must have taken 1, 2 and 3 as well (modules left = 32). (a)

5 nurses take module 3 (including the one who also did module 4) so 4 nurses took 12 modules. (b)

This means that 15 nurses must have taken the remaining 20 modules: the only way this is possible is if 10 took only 1, and 5 took 2. (c)

∴ the number of nurses taking module 2 is 5 + 4 + 1 = 10.

13 Biology class: B

This is very wordy, but is much simpler if you use a venn diagram (see numbered steps below).

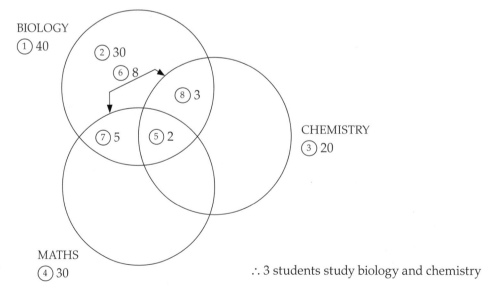

∴ 3 students study biology and chemistry

Bleach and asthma (14–17)

This is a long article, so look at the questions first; then you know what you are looking for when you read it.

14 B

B is the only factual statement from the article, and thus we can assume it to be accurate (that's why the question introduction says 'assuming the information in the article is accurate').

15 C

The article doesn't come to any conclusions regarding the link between cleaning products and asthma. Thus the other three statements are incorrect.

16 C

Easy: $10,000 \times 3 \times 3 = 90,000$

17 D

Be careful: in this age group, the majority of wheezing illness is *likely* to be established asthma. It is not a fact expressly mentioned by the article that children aged 9–11 suffer only from established asthma.

18 Damian and acceleration: D

This is easy.

$$a = \frac{\Delta S}{t}$$

$$A = \frac{150}{50} = 3$$

$$B = \frac{50}{50} = 1$$

$$C = \frac{10}{50} = 0.5$$

$$D = \frac{20}{5} = 4$$

Just be careful for D that you don't do $\frac{20}{50}$ (the speed reaches 20m/s at 5 seconds)

19 Charity donations: D

Pay careful attention to the instructions here. Note it says 'the *largest* donation that the third biggest charity can receive'. This means you have to give 4 and 5 the minimum (£21 and £20, respectively). This then leaves you with £359: £121, £120 and £118. Note that it can't be £119 as then you would have to give two amounts of £120, which is forbidden.

Boys and girls (20–22)

This looks horrible, but most of the adding up has been done for you.

20 B

$(420 - 80)/6 = 56.666$ (57)

21 B

Before move: $915/7 = 130.7$
After move: $(915 + 140)/8 = 131.6$
Difference $= 0.9$ (1)

22 C

Total rent $= 420 + 570 = 990$
$7.5\% = 5\% + 2.5\% = 49.50 + 24.75$
Total $= £1,064.25$

23 Wine stopper: 1.5π

Luckily the equation is given to you.
Work the volume out first.

$$6 \text{ cm cone} = \frac{1}{3}\pi r^2 h \qquad\qquad 3 \text{ cm cone} = \frac{1}{3}\pi r^2 h$$

$$= \frac{1}{3}\pi(0.25 \times 6) \qquad\qquad = \frac{1}{3}\pi(0.25 \times 3)$$

$$= \frac{1}{3}\pi \times 1.5 \qquad\qquad = \frac{1}{3}\pi \times 0.75$$

$$\text{Total} = \frac{1.5\pi + 0.75\pi}{3} = \frac{2.25\pi}{3}$$

$$\text{Mass} = \frac{2.25\pi}{3} \times 2 = \frac{4.5\pi}{3} = 1.5\pi$$

Chapter 14
Section 2: Scientific Knowledge and Applications

27 marks/30 minutes
Multiple choice or single best answer
No calculators allowed

On first glance, Section 2 of the BMAT looks to be the most difficult, due to its reliance on testing factual scientific and mathematical knowledge. Remember that the standard is only GCSE level, and the examiners are looking for this level of ability in your tackling scientific problems rather than, for example, a detailed knowledge of the periodic table. Do not worry if you have not studied the subject further than GCSE level and feel a little rusty: as each of the subject areas is similarly weighted, you are likely to make up in one area what you lose in another and, with practice, you will be surprised as to how much of your past studies you remember.

A number of subject areas will not be tested (as stated by BMAT). These are green plants as organisms (i.e. no photosynthesis); products from organic sources; products from metal ores and rocks; products from air; changes to the Earth and atmosphere; the Earth and beyond; and seismic waves. Looking at what is left in the GCSE syllabuses, combined with what aptitudes the BMAT aims to test, enables us to make an educated guess as to those subject areas that will be tested in the exam, including the following.

- Human biology
- Cells and cellular processes
- Basic maths – equations, fractions, multiplication, algebra (remember, no calculators)
- Basic physics equations
- Balancing chemical equations

Probably, these are all topics that you're studying or skills that you are using at the moment, but if you know you are weak in certain areas, such as your ability to do maths without a calculator or balancing equations, then get your old books out. Otherwise, what you really need to practise is time management – the challenge to obtain 27 marks in 30 minutes means you have to be speedy, accurate and decisive.

Again, note that there is no negative marking, so always give an answer. Work on the basis of 1 minute per question and, if you get stuck, move on after making a guess – you can return to it later if you have time. Remember that all the other candidates will be in the same boat as you time-wise, and an educated guess after reading a question will be better than going back through the paper in the last 30 seconds and filling in the questions you missed with wild guesses. There will also be lots of questions to which you know the answers immediately, and so this will give you a little more time for the questions you find more difficult.

It's usually best not to work out answers in your head as, under the pressure of the exam, mistakes are easily made and it also makes it difficult for you to check your answers if you have time on your hands later. The question paper can be used for all your working, but be aware that this is purely for your own benefit – you will only receive credit for answers correctly transferred and validly marked on the answer sheet.

Have a look at the past papers on the BMAT website to get an idea of what format the questions will take and what standard of knowledge you have to achieve. Below you will find some specimen questions to familiarise yourself with, together with their answers and solutions. These are just a flavour of the types of questions that could come up.

Some of the questions on the BMAT will be harder, some a little easier. Always look for the underlying rule or equation you have been taught that will allow you to solve the problem. Once you realise which equation or rule to apply, things will be a lot simpler. When you are familiar with the type of questions in Section 2, try the practice test at the end of this chapter and the ones on the BMAT website.

Example: maths

1   Simplify the following expression.
$$\frac{8a^3b \times 4a^2b^4}{2ab^2}$$

Answer
$$\frac{32a^5b^5}{2ab^2}$$
$$= 16a^4b^3$$

Remember, with powers you subtract when they are divided, and add when they are multiplied.

2 Give the value of A in the figure below.

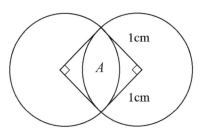

A $1 - \pi/4$

B $\pi - \frac{1}{2}$

C $1 - \pi/2$

D $\pi/2 - 1$

Answer

A bit tricky, but not if you realise that the area of a quarter of this circle is $\pi/4$ (πr^2 is the area of a circle – always look at the answers to give you a clue). The area of the square is 1 ($1 \times 1 = 1$). Within the square there are effectively two quarter circles – total area $\pi/2$ ($2 \times \pi/4$) – which overlap giving the area A:

$\pi/2 - A = 1$
$A = -1 + \pi/2$
$\therefore A = \pi/2 - 1$ (answer **D**)

Beware answer C, which results from incorrectly rearranging the equation. As always, look for the trick to the question, and then solve it quickly and accurately.

Example: chemistry

3 Calculate the relative formula mass, M_r, of ammonium sulphate, $(NH_4)_2SO_4$. ($N=14$, $H=1$, $S=32$, $O=16$).

Answer

$N=28$, $H=8$, $S=32$, $O=64$
$M_r = 132$.

Example: physics

4 A brick rests on a ledge and has a potential energy of 75J.
   When it falls, it hits the ground with a speed of $\sqrt{50}$ m/s.

   What is the mass of the brick?

   (Discount air resistance)

   A 3g

   B 30g

   C 300g

   D 3000g

Answer

Potential energy (PE) = kinetic energy (KE)

$$KE = \frac{1}{2} mv^2$$

$75 = 0.5 \times m \times (\sqrt{50})^2$

$75 = 25m \therefore m = 3$

As standard units are used, mass is in kilograms, therefore m = 3000g = D.

Example: biology

The diagram shows the inside of a human heart:

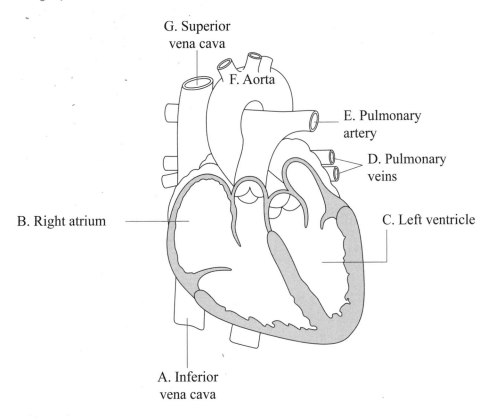

G. Superior
vena cava

F. Aorta

E. Pulmonary
artery

D. Pulmonary
veins

B. Right atrium

C. Left ventricle

A. Inferior
vena cava

5 Which vessel has the highest pressure during systole (contraction) of the heart?

6 Blood enters the inferior vena cava (A). Which of the following options best describes its subsequent route through the heart?

Ⓐ	A	G	B	E	D	C
Ⓑ	A	B	E	D	C	F
Ⓒ	A	B	E	C	D	F

Answers

5 This requires some knowledge of the human heart. Note that it says which *vessel*, not structure, has the highest pressure during systole.

The vessels to choose from are A, G, D, E and F. You should know that veins have lower pressures than arteries (with the exception of the pulmonary vein and artery). The left ventricle generates most of the blood pressure during systole, therefore the aorta (F) is the correct answer.

6   Blood flows from the right side of the heart to the left, via the lungs, then to the body via the aorta. Therefore B is the only correct option.

Section 2 practice test

Time allowed: 30 minutes

1 A tuning fork is being tested for accuracy:

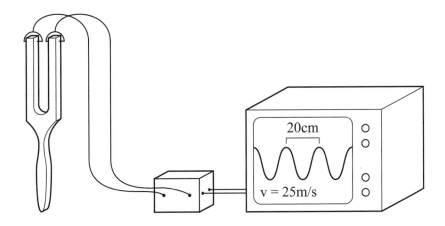

Tim records the velocity and wavelength as shown on the screen.

Give the frequency of the tuning fork's oscillation in hertz (Hz).

2 $5 \times 10^3 \div 2 \times 10^{-2}$.

Solve the equation above, giving your answer to the nearest whole number.

3 A solid block weighs 200 N and has the dimensions shown below.

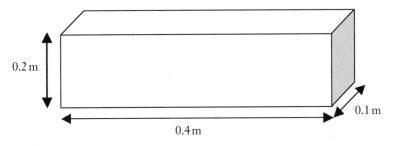

If the block can stand on any of its faces, what is the smallest pressure that the weight of the block will exert on the ground?

4   Below is a diagram depicting the knee-jerk reflex.

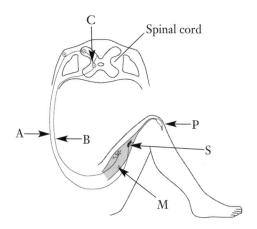

Place the letters in the correct order to describe the pathway of the stimulus and nerve impulse.

A S, M, B, C, A

B S, A, C, B, P

C P, S, A, C, B

D P, S, B, C, A

E P, B, C, A, S

5   Study the voltage–current graphs below.

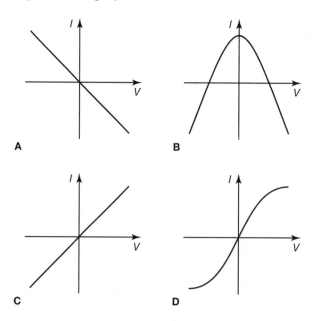

Which graph describes the resistance in

(i) a resistor;

(ii) a filament lamp?

6 A medical student takes a history from patient A, and constructs a family pedigree.

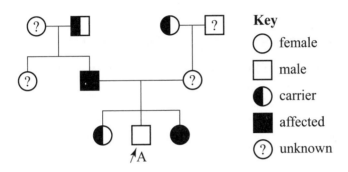

Key

◯ female

▢ male

◐ carrier

▪ affected

? unknown

What is the percentage probability that patient A is affected by the disease?

A   100%

B   75%

C   66%

D   50%

E   33%

F   25%

7 Which **two** of the following elements form compounds that are coloured?

A Copper

B Sodium

C Calcium

D Magnesium

E Iron

8 Which of the following is not found in the urine of a normal healthy adult. (Circle your answer).

uric acid
ammonia
urea
glucose
sodium chloride

9 Nitrogen (N_2) and hydrogen (H_2) react to make ammonia (NH_3).

A factory uses 28 tonnes of nitrogen in 2 hours. How much ammonia will be produced at maximal efficiency? (N=14, H=1)

10 In a particle accelerator a particle of mass 0.01 g travels at 400 m/s. If the particle comes to rest on a sensor in 1×10^{-4} seconds, what force is exerted on the sensor? Give your answer to the nearest whole number.

11

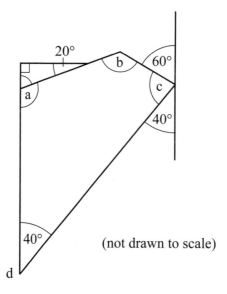

(not drawn to scale)

What is the value of angle b?

A   110°

B   130°

C   150°

D   160°

12 Rearrange the formula to make x the subject.

$$y - 2 = \sqrt{\frac{2}{x} + 1}$$

13 The diagram below shows a pregnant uterus.

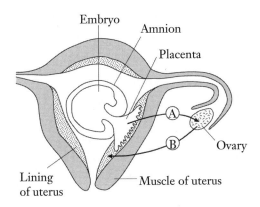

Circle the name of hormone A and draw a line under the name of hormone B.

Oestrogen   FSH   Adrenaline

Human chorionic gonadotrophin (HCG)

LH   Progesterone   Oestradiol

Questions 14–17 are based on the information below.

Ranil tests two substances, A and B, to find out what they contain. He knows that A is a sodium salt and that B is a chloride. His tests and results are shown overleaf.

Test	Result
Add dilute hydrochloric acid to solid A	A gas X is given off which turns limewater cloudy
Add sodium hydroxide solution to solid B and warm	A gas Y is given off which turns litmus paper blue

14 Select the name of gas X.

A   Chlorine

B   Carbon dioxide

C   Chloride

D   Hydrogen

15 Select the name of solid A.

    A   Sodium carbonate

    B   Sodium chloride

    C   Sodium hydroxide

    D   Sodium peroxide

16 Select the name of gas Y.

    A   Nitrous oxide

    B   Nitrogen

    C   Hydrogen

    D   Ammonia

17 Select the name of solid B.

    A   Nitrogen chloride

    B   Nitrogen hydroxide

    C   Nitrous oxide

    D   Ammonium chloride

18 Which of the following factor pairs describe the equation $c^2 - 3c - 10$?

    A $(c + 2)(c + 5)$

    B $(c - 2)(c + 5)$

    C $(c - 2)(c - 5)$

    D $(c + 2)(c - 5)$

19 The line below has an intersection with the line $y = 2x + 4$.

Where do the graphs intersect? (Give your answer as co-ordinates.)

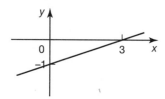

Questions 20–22 are based on the following diagram and labels.

Label the diagram of the thorax using the labels provided. They may be used once, more than once, or not at all.

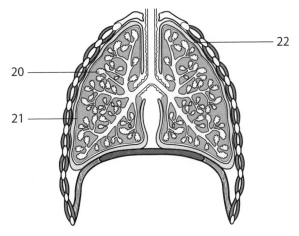

A   Bronchiole

B   Visceral pleura

C   Liver

D   Trachea

E   Rib

F   Lobe

G   Blood

H   Bone

I   Alveolus

J   Parietal pleura

K   Intercostal muscle

L   Diaphragm

23 Look at the table of hormones involved in glucose homeostasis. Which combinations of hormones would be seen in a healthy individual?

	Blood sugar	Insulin	Glucagon
A	↓	↑	↑
B	↑	↓	↑
C	↓	↓	↑
D	↑	↑	↓
E	↓	↓	↓

24 Which of the following formulae for ethanol is correct?

A C_2H_6

B CH_2OH

C C_2H_5OH

D $C_2H_5OH_2$

Section 2 practice test: answers

Question number	Correct response	Comments	Marks
1	125 Hz		1
2	250,000		1
3	2,500 Pa		1
4	C		1
5	(i) C (ii) D	Both for 1 mark	1
6	D		1
7	A and E	Both correct for 1 mark	1
8	Glucose		1
9	34 tonnes		1
10	40 N	1 mark for units	2
11	B		1
12	$x = \dfrac{2}{(y - 3)(y - 1)}$		1
13	A = HCG; B = progesterone	Both correct for 1 mark	1
14	B		1
15	A		1
16	D		1
17	D		1
18	D		1
19	(−3, −2)		1
20	I		1
21	B		1
22	J		1
23	C and D		2
24	C		1

Section 2 practice test: explanation of answers

1 Tuning fork: 125 Hz

velocity (V) = frequency(f) × wavelength(λ)

V = f × λ (where velocity is in m/s, frequency is in Hz and wavelength is in m)

25 = f × 0.2 (note 20 cm = 0.2 m)

$f = \dfrac{25}{0.2} = 125\,\text{Hz}$

2 Exponents: 250 000

$\dfrac{5 \times 10^3}{2 \times 10^{-2}} = 2.5 \times 10^5$ (remember to add the powers, and negative denominators become positive)

$2.5 \times 10^5 = 250\,000$

3 Solid block: 2,500 Pa
They would probably give you a choice of answers for this one, but it may be more fun to work it out yourself. The smallest pressure will result from the block resting on its largest area:
0.4 × 0.2 = 0.08
Pressure = Force/Area
Pressure = 200/0.08 = 2,500 Pa – always remember your units.

4 Knee jerk: C
Patella tap (P) is sensed by the sensory nerves in the muscle (S) which is then relayed via the afferent nerves (A) to the spinal cord (C) and then down the efferent nerves (B) to the muscle (M), which contracts to move the leg.

5 Resistance graphs: C, D
   (i)   Resistors have a steady resistance producing a straight-line positive graph
         (R = V/I)
   (ii) Filament lamps are non-ohmic – their resistance increases as they heat up, also
         in a positive manner.

6 Family tree: D.
This is a recessive trait, like cystic fibrosis, or sickle cell disease.
The mother of A must be a carrier to produce an affected sister.
No children will be unaffected; they have a 50% chance of being a carrier and a 50% chance of being affected.

7 Coloured compounds: A and E
A knowledge one here. Think back to your practical sessions or, if stumped, then think sensibly – copper and iron are both coloured metals.

8 Kidney: glucose

The kidney acts as an ultrafiltration and dialysis system – glucose is too large to cross the normal renal capsule.

9 Ammonia factory: 34 tonnes

First, write down the equation.

N_2 $+ 3H_2$ $= 2NH_3$
1 mole   :   3 moles   :   2 moles
$2 \times 14 = 28$ g   : $3 \times 2 = 6$ g   :   34 g
28 tonnes   :   6 tonnes   :   34 tonnes.

Take care with these sorts of equations. There weren't any charges to worry about, but there could easily be in a different question.

10 Particle accelerator: 40 N

$f = ma$: $a = \Delta s/t = 400/1 \times 10^{-4}$
$f = 1 \times 10^{-5} \times 400/1 \times 10^{-4}$ (remember mass is in kg)
$= 40$ N (don't forget the units)

11 Angles: B.

Remember angles in a triangle and along a line add up to 180°, and angles in a quadrilateral add up to 360°.

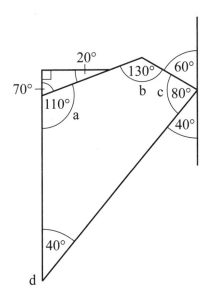

12 Rearrangement: $x = \dfrac{2}{(y-3)(y-1)} + 1$

$$y - 2 = \sqrt{\tfrac{2}{x} + 1}$$

$$(y-2)^2 = \frac{2}{x} + 1$$

$$y^2 - 4y + 4 = \frac{2}{x} + 1$$

$$y^2 - 4y + 3 = \frac{2}{x}$$

$$x = \frac{2}{y^2 - 4y + 3}$$

$$\therefore x = \frac{2}{(y-3)(y-1)}$$

13 Pregnant uterus: A = HCG, B = progesterone

HCG is secreted from the implanted blastocyst to inhibit further ovulation, while progesterone is secreted by the ovary to maintain the lining of the womb and to support the process of implantation. Unfortunately this is another knowledge-based question, although you could probably have a good guess from the answers supplied. If you have no idea of the answer, then the best thing is to guess and move on rapidly: spend the time on some of the questions that require you to work out the answer.

14–17 Chemical reactions: B, A, D, D

Carbon dioxide turns limewater cloudy.

Only a carbonate produces CO_2 when it reacts with acid.

Ammonia gas turns damp litmus paper blue (it is alkaline).

Ammonia gas is produced from ammonium chloride when mixed with sodium hydroxide.

18 Factorising quadratics: D

This is a very quick and easy question. Just make sure you don't get yourself confused between B and D.

19 Equations of lines: (–3, –2)

The equation of the line is

$$y = mx + c$$

$$y = \frac{1}{3}x - 1$$

Intersection: $\dfrac{1}{3}x - 1 = 2x + 4$

$$-\frac{5}{3}x = 5$$

$$-5x = 15 \therefore x = -3$$

$$2x + 4 = y$$

$$-6 + 4 = y \therefore y = -2$$

20–22 Apparatus of breathing: I, B, J

The only mistake you might make is confusing the visceral and parietal pleura. Remember 'visceral' is a word for organs, so the visceral pleura abuts the lungs.

23 Insulin and glucagon: C and D

Remember that the job of insulin is to decrease blood sugar by taking it into cells, whereas glucagon releases stored insulin into the blood.

24 Ethanol: C

The formula is C_2H_5OH.

Chapter 15
Section 3: Writing Task

Choose one of three questions
30 minutes inclusive of planning and writing
Only one-page response allowed

Most BMAT candidates neglect to prepare for the final section of the test, either sacrificing the time for more preparation on the first two sections or believing that it isn't the type of task you can prepare for. If you have already looked at the questions in the specimen papers, you will have realised that they are very different from the type of factual essay you are used to writing in biology exams. Indeed, they seem more at home in a philosophy admissions exam than the BMAT.

However, the very fact that Section 3 is different from your normal A-level essays means that you should invest time in preparing for it – this section of the BMAT has been included specifically to test the skills that will be vital for your biomedical degree. An excellent answer on this section of the BMAT will demonstrate that you can:

- recognise and resolve conflict;
- formulate and provide valid support for logical arguments;
- consider alternative explanations for difficult ideas.

Looked at in this way, Section 3 suddenly seems a lot more relevant to your application than you probably thought it was. After you are happy with the question format and answer strategy of the first two sections of the BMAT, you should turn your attention to some proper preparation for the Writing Task. Time spent in preparation will reap bigger rewards than practising the same old multiple-choice questions again and again until you can do them in your sleep.

In order to prepare for the Writing Task, it is best to try to get your hands on the broadsheet newspapers and to keep up to date with the topical medical and ethico-legal debates. For example, there are always debates about whether the NHS should fund the purchase of unproven drug treatment regimens (think about the benefit for one versus the cost to many) or about court cases regarding ventilating terminally ill patients (which have to balance the right to life against the right to have a peaceful and private death). This isn't really the type of research that you can do on the night before the BMAT exam: not only will effective preparation allow you to incorporate convincing examples into your essays but it will also help you to think critically and to challenge information that is presented to you.

The best way you can prepare for this section of the BMAT is to invest in a notebook, divide each page in two and write down 'for' and 'against' arguments for each biological/medical/ethical/legal debate that you come across. Not only will this help you to clarify your ideas but it will also provide you with a fantastic revision prompt for the night before the BMAT. Although the issues you choose may not be asked about explicitly, you will build up a large library of examples, allowing you to answer the BMAT question that most appeals to you, as opposed to the only one that you could write two lines about.

As an added incentive, any time spent in researching for the BMAT won't be wasted. These sorts of ethical and biomedical debates make ideal interview topics, and interviewers will give credit to a candidate who can back up his or her arguments with elegant and relevant examples, compared with one who justifies his or her response with 'I just think it's wrong'.

However, in order to turn the brilliant examples you will collect into sparkling essays, you need to practise essay planning. Below you will find a breakdown of a BMAT-style Section 3 question that describes how you should order and arrange your essay and how to incorporate scientific examples effectively. Also included in this chapter is a Section 3 practice test, complete with suggested answers in the form of spider diagrams. You will appreciate that every answer is different, and it is how you incorporate your ideas into your essays that counts in the end (and in your score). If you work through these examples and practise arranging your answers as described, you can feel confident that you are effectively prepared for the final section. It cannot be emphasised enough that you will receive a score directly proportional to the time and effort you invest in preparation, so make sure you prioritise wisely.

It is also worth having a look at the BMAT marking criteria for Section 3, available on the BMAT website. From this, you will see that there are separate marking criteria for quality of content and quality of English. Before you get stuck in, consider that the final section is as much a test of how well you can follow instructions as of what you can actually write. The following points may seem obvious, but the low average scores for the BMAT Section 3 suggest that perhaps they aren't.

Read the questions carefully

Take the time to read all the question choices and to decide which one of the choice of four questions you could answer the best. You would be surprised at the number of candidates who simply choose the first question on the paper (often in sheer relief that they can actually answer it). The question that seems impossible at first may offer a wealth of possibility on the second reading.

Plan your essay

You must always write an essay plan. Half an hour is plenty of time for you to write a single page of A4, so I would advise spending ten minutes of the time choosing your question carefully, and planning and thinking of examples. There is nothing worse than getting half-way through your answer and realising that you have completely run out of points to make, leading to your repeating yourself or leaving half of the answer space empty. More frequently, candidates run out of time or space on the sheet and have to miss out the conclusion, which is as vital a part of your answer as the examples that you give.

Planning an essay allows you to write an effective introduction and conclusion: there is no need to use the age-old trick of leaving a space at the start of your essay to write the introduction at the end if you have planned your entire answer in advance.

Answer the question

Always answer the question(s) asked. You have probably heard this a hundred times before but, unfortunately, too many candidates run off at a tangent and neglect to answer the question in hand (which scores them few or no marks). If the examiners don't ask about it, they don't want to hear about it. That's not to say that you can't cleverly draw pre-prepared examples into your answer, but be aware that, unless you explicitly answer the question, and answer all parts, your answer will be marked little higher than an incomplete or absent answer. Try ticking the questions off as you answer them in your plan to ensure you incorporate all of them into your answer.

Avoid bias

Consider both sides of the question and/or argument. The examiners deliberately set questions that do not have a definite or right answer, which means that you have to present both sides of the argument. If you read some of the sample answers on the website you will notice that, often, they aren't very balanced and, as a result, they seem rather shallow and uninformed.

Include a couple of points in support of the argument and a couple against, and follow them up with your own opinions on the matter. Even if the question seems to ask just for your opinion, you must always present evidence as to why you think this in the form of examples, and always demonstrate that you have considered alternative answers to the problem. It is very important to show the examiner that you do not harbour any unfair prejudices – you do want them to let you into medical, dental or vet school after all.

Answer within the space provided

Use all the space provided but no more. Following instructions is important, and they have provided you with just one sheet of ruled A4 so that you write no more and no less. However, each year failure to plan the essay adequately causes many students to run out of space and to torture the examiner with teeny-tiny mouse-size script snaking its way up the margins, over the page and on to the desk. Unlike in AS exams, the examiners aren't impressed by the expanse of your knowledge and will definitely mark you down for your failure to follow instructions and demonstration of poor planning. An excellent answer can be produced easily within the confines of one page, so when the lines stop, so do you.

First of all, let's consider how we would go about tackling some BMAT-type questions.

In the scientific world, advancements can only be made if mistakes are allowed to happen.

Explain what you think is meant by this statement: Can scientific advancements be made without mistakes being made first? What do you think determines whether a scientific outcome is a mistake or advancement?

Note that there are lots of 'mini-questions' in the main question, aimed at helping you to consider all aspects of your answer. The best way to cover these is to use them as the basis of your introduction, main body and conclusion. Also, make sure you take note of the trigger words in each question, which you may find helpful to underline.

Explain what <u>you</u> think is meant by this statement.

This is the perfect opportunity to grab the examiner's attention and acts as your introduction to your essay. Don't be afraid to state the obvious – they don't use trick questions. Below is one possible answer.

Scientific advancements arise as the result of many years of study and research and, in order to find the correct answer to a problem, you often have to make many mistakes first.

Although this is a good start, the answer fails to incorporate a personal touch (they are asking what you think after all) and also does not explain why mistakes have to be made (as opposed to the fact that they are just a part of research). A better answer would be something like the following.

I believe that this statement is describing the fact that, in science, there is no proof: a hypothesis can only be demonstrated to be wrong. In order to move forward, we have to demonstrate that all other theories are wrong. One way that this happens is through the process of making mistakes, and hence making mistakes becomes a vital part of scientific discovery.

This forms a concise and elegant introduction to your essay and will also lead nicely into some examples. It gives a flavour of what is to come and should tie in well with a conclusion. It also shows that you have planned your answer: it is often only when you start to plan examples for and against an argument that you realise what the original statement means.

Can scientific advancements be made without mistakes being made first?

This question should form the basis of the main body of your essay. It is just asking to be answered with lots of examples for and against (after you have done a few of this type of question, you will realise that they are all the same and the mini-questions will practically walk you through your answer).

It is probably easier to think of examples where mistakes had to be made for scientific advancement to be possible, and then to consider examples when they didn't. It may be that you find one half of the argument much harder than the other, and this will probably point you in the direction of what your conclusion should be.

This question is asking for scientific examples, but even if the question doesn't explicitly ask, try to choose examples that have some relevance to medicine or biomedical science – this is the BMAT after all. The best examples you could choose are the ones that could be argued both ways.

Scientific advancements with mistakes.

- *Drug testing*: at all stages of drug trials scientists are looking for side-effects and problems with the drugs. If there are, this means the drug is not fit for its designed purpose, which means there has been a 'mistake'. New drugs can only be developed by learning from these mistakes and refining the drug formula. Specific example: drug trial for Thalidomide led to the recognition that isomeric forms of drugs can be dangerous.
- *Transplants*: in the past, organ transplantation often led to rejection – the ultimate failure or 'mistake'. This prompted scientists to research why rejection was happening, leading to the scientific advancement of tissue-matching donor organs with recipients.

Scientific advancements without mistakes.

- *Fleming's discovery of penicillin*: Fleming discovered penicillin growing in his laboratory; the drug is still used today.
- *Early Renaissance scientists dissecting human cadavers pushed forward the knowledge of anatomy*: by actually observing the structures they could make no mistakes in describing them, although they did not understand all the functions of the organs or the changes that occurred at death.

What do you think determines whether a scientific outcome is a mistake or an advancement?

This question is asking you to write a conclusion, incorporating the points you have already made. An average BMAT candidate will either neglect to answer this question properly or give an inarticulate answer. You should concentrate on two or three points you can use to draw everything together.

- Expected or not expected.
- Future work.
- Limits of current knowledge.

Here you have three examples of what determines whether a scientific outcome is a mistake or advancement. State them categorically and use your existing examples to back them up – this adds to the feeling that you have planned an integrated essay.

There are a number of factors that determine whether a scientific outcome is a mistake or advancement. First, it depends whether the outcome is expected or not expected. If, during a drug trial, it is expected that a reaction will occur, then if this reaction happens the outcome will add to scientific knowledge and become an advancement. If a reaction is not expected it could be classed as a mistake, but often investigation into why this mistake happened results in scientific advancement.

Secondly, it is often only future discoveries that confirm the status of a scientific outcome: there are always examples of fortuitous discoveries in science, such as Fleming discovering penicillin growing in his laboratory. However, it was only through future work, involving mistakes, that this discovery became a practical scientific advancement.

Lastly, the limits of current knowledge determine our perception of whether it is a mistake or advancement. It is only when the correct solution is reached that we realise where we had been going wrong, such as in the knowledge of organ rejection. It is only in retrospect and with the knowledge acquired from such experiments that we can classify them as mistakes. Therefore scientific progress relies on outcomes that are both mistakes and advances.

Notice how the questions are summarised in the last line of the answer. This is a trick you will all be familiar with from GCSE English, and it works here too in leading the examiner to believe you have answered the question more directly and concisely than you may have actually done. Just be careful that you don't rely on it solely as a conclusion: the examiners are familiar with this trick and will award you nothing for your efforts.

Have a look at the answer written by previous BMAT students on the website. Try to count the number of points raised and the examples given. Often even the answers that receive the best marks only contain a few examples, so you can see how much they will do for your score. If you doubt that you could produce such a coherent argument, incorporating ready-prepared ideas will be much more effective than trying to think up examples on the spot. Also remember that exam conditions have the effect of making you write faster, so you don't need to worry about incorporating all your examples in the time allowed.

Now that you have seen how to break down a question into its component parts, you should practise answering sample questions yourself, ensuring that all the questions are answered and that your essay hangs together well. After you have done a few questions you will realise that they all follow the same basic outline, with the multiple sub-questions acting as prompts for your introduction, main arguments and conclusion.

Once you are familiar with the approach to essay writing, rather than spending your preparation time in writing out page-long answers, I suggest you prepare spider diagrams to generate essay plans. This also has the benefit of being quick and easy to do in the BMAT exam itself, allowing you to draw links and contrasts between your arguments and to stay focused on the question. You can also tick off the points and examples as you progress through your essay, which helps significantly with time management.

Have a look at the example spider diagrams for the sample questions below to gain an understanding of how they can be used effectively. If you feel a bit unsure about essay writing, then you could use the example spider diagrams as a basis for your practice essays so that you can get a feel for how much of the contents you can incorporate into your essay in the 20–25 minutes of writing time you have during the exam. When you are confident in turning essay plans into great essays, then your remaining preparation can focus on generating spider diagrams and collecting examples.

At the end of this chapter I have included three more specimen tests for you to use either for spider diagram or essay practice, and you can also use the BMAT past papers as a basis for your spider diagrams. If you do use the BMAT past papers, remember that, while the style of the questions changes very little, the actual question topics will change, so it isn't wise to spend too much time preparing answers and examples for the specific questions in the past papers.

Example essay questions

1 **'Stop moaning! The pain is there to help you!'**

What does the above statement imply? Give examples that illustrate how pain can be beneficial and others that illustrate the opposite. How can you explain the differences in the function of pain?

2   **In the modern age of science, the laws of natural selection no longer apply to humans.**

What do you understand by the statement above? Can you suggest examples where natural selection still applies and examples where it does not? What factors affect whether natural selection applies to a species?

3   **Health and disease are points along a continuum, rather than separate states.**

Explain what the meaning of this statement is. Do you agree with this statement? Advance arguments in support of and in opposition to this statement. What determines the balance between health and disease?

4   **The Animal Welfare Act (2006) makes owners and keepers responsible for ensuring that the welfare needs of their animals are met.**

What welfare needs do animals have? Are there any possible conflicts between upholding the welfare needs of animals and the rights of owners/keepers? Should animals have the same rights as humans?

Example essay questions: suggested answers

1 'Stop moaning! The pain is there to help you!'

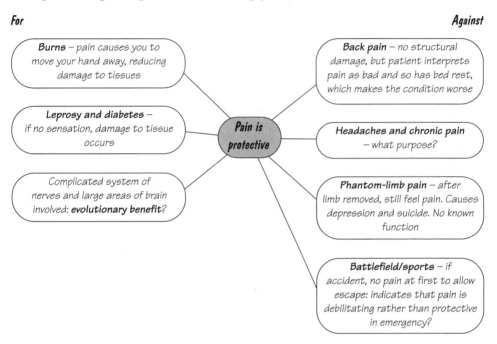

For   *Against*

Burns – pain causes you to move your hand away, reducing damage to tissues

Leprosy and diabetes – if no sensation, damage to tissue occurs

Complicated system of nerves and large areas of brain involved: **evolutionary benefit?**

Pain is protective

Back pain – no structural damage, but patient interprets pain as bad and so has bed rest, which makes the condition worse

Headaches and chronic pain – what purpose?

Phantom-limb pain – after limb removed, still feel pain. Causes depression and suicide. No known function

Battlefield/sports – if accident, no pain at first to allow escape: indicates that pain is debilitating rather than protective in emergency?

Statement implies

Pain is largely assumed by lay people to be a negative and harmful process, but the fact that complex pain pathways and mechanisms exist in humans may indicate it is protective and therefore of evolutionary benefit. The statement is also indicating that it is of a day-to-day benefit.

How can you explain the differences?

- Lack of knowledge (e.g. headache may serve some protective function).
- Pain may be so vital that mechanisms are 'hard-wired' into brain and independent of limbs, etc. (e.g. phantom limb pain).
- Psychological aspect of pain: different people in different circumstances feel the same pain differently (e.g. a broken leg on the sports field may hurt less than if someone attacks you).
- Different situations: pain sensation in the feet is wanted – lost in diabetes – but chronic pain that appears to serve no purpose is unwanted.

2   **In the modern age of science, the laws of natural selection no longer apply to humans.**

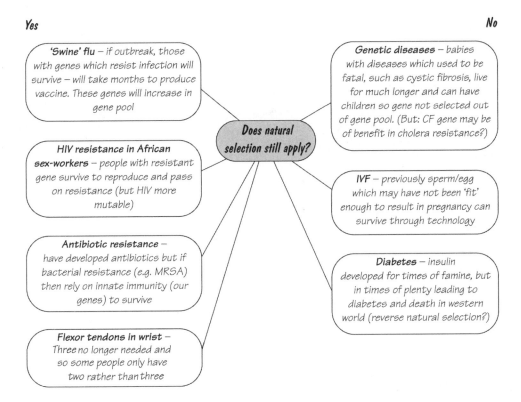

Yes

'**Swine' flu** – *if outbreak, those with genes which resist infection will survive – will take months to produce vaccine. These genes will increase in gene pool*

HIV resistance in African sex-workers – *people with resistant gene survive to reproduce and pass on resistance (but HIV more mutable)*

Antibiotic resistance – *have developed antibiotics but if bacterial resistance (e.g. MRSA) then rely on innate immunity (our genes) to survive*

Flexor tendons in wrist – *Three no longer needed and so some people only have two rather than three*

Does natural selection still apply?

No

Genetic diseases – *babies with diseases which used to be fatal, such as cystic fibrosis, live for much longer and can have children so gene not selected out of gene pool. (But: CF gene may be of benefit in cholera resistance?)*

IVF – *previously sperm/egg which may have not been 'fit' enough to result in pregnancy can survive through technology*

Diabetes – *insulin developed for times of famine, but in times of plenty leading to diabetes and death in western world (reverse natural selection?)*

Statement means

Natural selection = Darwin's theory of 'survival of the fittest' – i.e. those best adapted to their environment survive and pass on their genes. In the modern age these rules may not apply due to medical and scientific support which effectively adapts the environment for us.

What factors affect whether natural selection applies?

- Environment – the difference with humans is that we can change our environment to a large extent. But when the environment changes, it takes time for us to adapt.
- Reproduction – now assisted (e.g. IVF: can increase disease genes).
- Mixing of gene pool.
- Mutation rate – much slower in humans – we have evolved mechanisms to prevent DNA mutation.
- Time – generation time is much longer in humans; see changes slowly.

3   Health and disease are points along a continuum, rather than separate states.

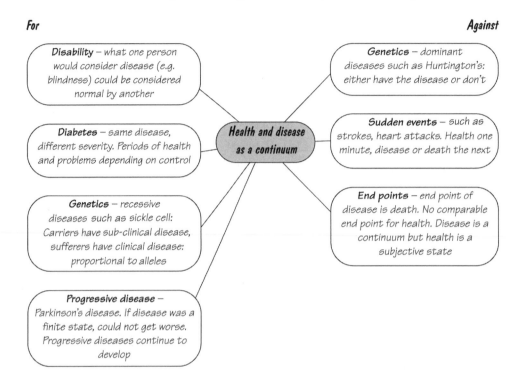

Statement means

Health is often considered as the absence of disease. Hence one cannot exist without the other. It is the loss of full health that, for most people, constitutes disease, and the impact of this loss of health can vary greatly between individuals.

What determines the balance between health and disease?

- Individual perception
- Perception of society
- Medical advances 'normalise' some diseases so they seem less severe (e.g. diabetes)
- Nature and nurture

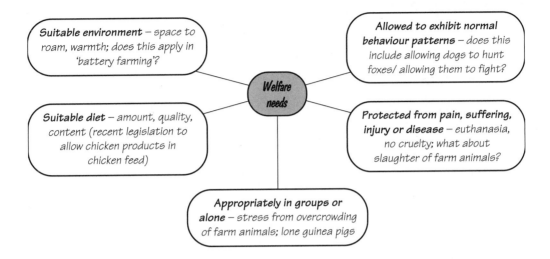

4 **The Animal Welfare Act (2006): Owners' and keepers' responsibility**

Remember to think about both pets and livestock!

Should animals have the same rights as humans?

Should the right to life without cruelty be universal?

Should animals have the right to be protected from suffering? Does this include slaughtering animals, and the issue of euthanasia which is not possible in humans?

Now you have some idea of how to break down the questions and understand how to use a spider diagram, have a go at creating spider diagrams and writing essays using the practice tests at the end of this chapter. There are no correct answers, but enlist your family, friends and teachers to help look over your essay plans and essays – after all, you want to try to achieve the broadest perspective on your outlook, and they will be able to suggest ideas and examples that you may never have thought of.

Although it is tempting to concentrate on the questions to which you already know you could give a good answer, attempt some of the ones that look less attractive. In the exam it will seem like all the questions are horrible and impossible to answer so, if you practise answering some that you find more difficult at this stage, you will be well prepared by the time you come to take the BMAT.

Section 3 practice test

Time allowed: 30 minutes

Practice test A

YOU MUST ANSWER <u>ONLY</u> ONE OF THE FOLLOWING QUESTIONS

1 'Extreme remedies are very appropriate for extreme diseases' – Hippocrates, 'Aphorisms'

'There are some remedies worse than the disease' – Publilius Syrus

Which of these statements do you agree with? Give some examples in support of these arguments. How can we reconcile these differing aspects of remedies?

2 'A cost to an individual can be justified by a benefit to the group.'

Do you agree with this hypothesis? Outline arguments in support of and in opposition to this statement. What factors influence the rights of an individual over that of the group?

3 'You can only believe in what you know to be true.'

What relevance does this statement have to scientific thought? Advance an argument against this idea. What other factors influence scientific belief?

4 'As medicine advances, so too does the bill.'

What do you think is meant by this statement? Can you give examples of where this statement is correct/incorrect? What factors affect the costs of medical science?

END OF TEST

Practice test B

YOU MUST ANSWER ONLY <u>ONE</u> OF THE FOLLOWING QUESTIONS

1 **'The right to life carries with it the right to death.'**

Discuss the implications of this statement. In what circumstances would you agree with this idea, and in what circumstances would you disagree? What factors would influence the possession of such rights?

2 **'If a man will begin with certainties, he shall end in doubts, but if he will be content to begin with doubts, he shall end in certainties' – Francis Bacon**

What do you interpret this statement to mean? Can you think of any examples where he is right? Can you ever know something for certain?

3 **'Medicine is an art form rather than a scientific discipline.'**

Do you agree with this statement? In what ways could medicine be considered an art form, and in what ways could it be considered a scientific discipline?

4 **'A scientific man ought to have no wishes, no affections, – a mere heart of stone' – Charles Darwin**

What does Darwin mean by this statement? Do you think he is right? Give examples in science, human or animal medicine to support your answer.

END OF TEST

Practice test C

YOU MUST ANSWER ONLY <u>ONE</u> OF THE FOLLOWING QUESTIONS

1 **'The ability to laugh is what makes us human.'**

What different meanings could this statement have? Advance arguments for the genetic versus the environmental effect on our personality development.

2 **'All perceived benefits carry with them a known risk.'**

Discuss, with examples, whether this statement is true. How could we resolve the conflict between benefit and harm?

3 **'Genes control our lives.'**

Explain what the statement above means. Advance an argument in support of and in opposition to the statement. How can we identify the role that genes play in our lives?

4 **'That knowledge which is popular is not scientific.'**

What do you think the author means by this statement? Give examples of scientific advancements which have been popular and/or unpopular. How can we achieve public understanding of scientific principles?

END OF TEST

Chapter 16
After the BMAT

Depending on the university you applied to and the style of interview, you may be asked about your essay when you go for interview, as BMAT sends each of the universities a copy of your Section 3 script along with your marks for Sections 1 and 2. The interviewers won't ask you about spelling and grammar, but they may ask you about your essay, especially if they thought it was well written or had some good ideas (which should be the case after all your hard work). They will always give you a copy of your answer, but it's always useful to have had a refresher read beforehand. Therefore it is advisable to spend 10 minutes after you come out of the exam jotting down the spider diagram you used for your essay, along with the major examples. Not only will this keep your mind off which questions your friends got right and you didn't, but it will also serve as an aide-mémoire when you are preparing for your interview, because it is almost guaranteed you won't remember anything about your BMAT test by the time your interview comes around a month or two later. It may well be that you never hear anything further about your BMAT exam, but 10 minutes spent now will at least stop you worrying about the possibility of having to talk about your essay later on.

Good luck for the big day. If you have prepared to the best of your ability, then you can be satisfied that you will fulfil your potential, however tough the exam. This effort and the skills that you learn will stand you in good stead for your future career.

Also Available.....

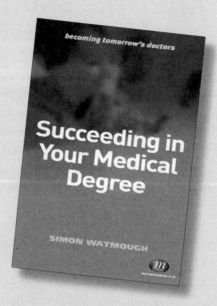

The first title in an exciting new series *Becoming Tomorrow's Doctors* specifically written to help students to succeed in their medical careers.

ISBN: 9780857253972, Price: £17.00

To order, visit **www.learningmatters.co.uk** or call 0845 230 9000